OXFORD MEDICAL PUBLICATIONS

Vascular Surgery

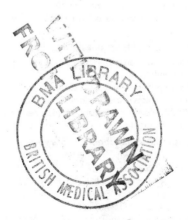

Published and forthcoming Oxford Specialist Handbooks

General Oxford Specialist Handbooks

A Resuscitation Room Guide (Banerjee and Hargreaves)

Oxford Specialist Handbooks in End of Life Care

Cardiology: From advanced disease to bereavement (Beattie, Connelly, and Watson eds.)

Nephrology: From advanced disease to bereavement (Brown, Chambers, and Eggeling)

Oxford Specialist Handbooks in Anaesthesia

Cardiac Anaesthesia (Barnard and Martin eds.)

Neuroanaesthesia (Nathanson and Moppett eds.)

Obstetric Anaesthesia (Clyburn, Collis, Harries, and Davies eds.)

Paediatric Anaesthesia (Doyle ed.)

Oxford Specialist Handbooks in Cardiology

Cardiac Catheterization and Coronary Angiography (Mitchell, Leeson, West, and Banning)

Pacemakers and ICDs (Timperley, Leeson, Mitchell, and Betts eds.)

Echocardiography (Leeson, Mitchell, and Becher eds.)

Heart Failure (Gardner, McDonagh, and Walker)

Nuclear Cardiology (Kelion, Loong, and Sabharwal)

Oxford Specialist Handbooks in Neurology

Epilepsy (Alarcon, Nashaf, Cross, and Nightingale)

Parkinson's Disease and Other Movement Disorders (Edwards, Bhatia, Quinn, and Swinn)

Oxford Specialist Handbooks in Paediatrics

Paediatric Gastroenterology, Hepatology, and Nutrition (Beattie, Dhawan, and Puntis eds.)

Paediatric Nephrology (Rees, Webb, and Brogan)

Paediatric Neurology (Forsyth and Newton eds.)

Paediatric Oncology and Haematology (Bailey and Skinner eds.)

Paediatric Radiology (Johnson, Williams, and Foster)

Oxford Specialist Handbooks in Surgery

Hand Surgery (Warwick)

Neurosurgery (Samandouras)

Otolaryngology and Head and Neck Surgery (Corbridge and Warner)

Plastic and Reconstructive Surgery (Giele and Cassell eds.)

Renal Transplantation (Talbot)

Urology (Reynard, Sullivan, Turner, Feneley, Armenakas, and Mark eds.)

Vascular Surgery (Hands, Murphy, Sharp, and Ray-Chaudhuri)

Oxford Specialist Handbooks
in Surgery

Vascular Surgery

Edited by

Linda Hands
Clinical Reader in Surgery
Nuffield Department of Surgery
University of Oxford, John Radcliffe Hospital
Oxford, UK

Michael Murphy
Clinical Lecturer in Surgery
Nuffield Department of Surgery
University of Oxford, John Radcliffe Hospital
Oxford, UK

Michael Sharp
Locum Consultant Surgeon
Aberdeen Royal Infirmary
Aberdeen, UK

and

Simon Ray-Chaudhuri
Consultant Surgeon
Milton Keynes General Hospital
Buckinghamshire, UK

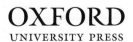

OXFORD
UNIVERSITY PRESS

OXFORD

UNIVERSITY PRESS

Great Clarendon Street, Oxford OX2 6DP

Oxford University Press is a department of the University of Oxford.
It furthers the University's objective of excellence in research, scholarship,
and education by publishing worldwide in

Oxford New York

Auckland Cape Town Dar es Salaam Hong Kong Karachi
Kuala Lumpur Madrid Melbourne Mexico City Nairobi
New Delhi Shanghai Taipei Toronto

With offices in

Argentina Austria Brazil Chile Czech Republic France Greece
Guatemala Hungary Italy Japan Poland Portugal Singapore
South Korea Switzerland Thailand Turkey Ukraine Vietnam

Oxford is a registered trade mark of Oxford University Press
in the UK and in certain other countries

Published in the United States
by Oxford University Press Inc., New York

British Library Cataloguing in Publication Data

Data available

Library of Congress Cataloging in Publication Data

Data available

Typeset by Newgen Imaging Systems (P) Ltd., Chennai, India
Printed in Italy
on acid-free paper by
Legoprint S.p.A.

ISBN 978-0-19-920308-6 (Flexicover: alk.paper)

10 9 8 7 6 5 4 3 2 1

Preface

Vascular surgery is an evolving speciality, which has to embrace the current developments in interventional vascular radiology whilst looking to future changes in training that may encompass more of the 'medical' aspects of vascular disease. Nevertheless, open surgical techniques still play a large role in the management of the vascular patient and will do so for some time to come. The vascular surgeon needs to be a physician who can operate, but who also knows when to operate.

This book is designed to give detailed guidance on the work up, perioperative management, and operative details for patients undergoing vascular surgery. It concentrates on open procedures but includes details on endovascular aortic aneurysm stenting and offers endovascular alternatives to surgical intervention where they exist. These details reflect the practice of the chapter author; they are not intended as the only possible approach and in many cases there are alternatives. OPCS 4.3 (2007) codes are included for each procedure so that they become familiar to the surgical team in an environment where accurate recording of activity is becoming essential.

The book is designed primarily for the training grade doctor to carry in their pocket on the ward, in clinic, and in the operating theatre. It is designed for quick reference and rapid reading and will help resolve uncertainties on the ward and prepare the trainee for their role in theatre, whether as prime operator or as assistant. It should also be helpful to F1 and F2 doctors involved in the care of vascular patients by providing background on the disease, details of ward management, and an idea of what happens in theatre. The trainee vascular anaesthetist will find useful detail not only on anaesthetic management but also on what is going on at the other end of the table. Similarly, trainee interventional radiologists, vascular nurses, and vascular technologists will all find that a broader appreciation of vascular patient management can be obtained from this book.

Linda Hands
Michael Murphy
Michael Sharp
Simon Ray-Chaudhuri
January 2007.

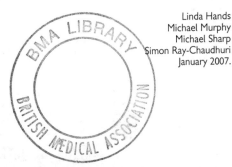

Contents

Detailed contents

Contributors

Mr Ashok Handa
Nuffield Department of Surgery,
John Radcliffe Hospital, Oxford
Chapter 5: Non-operative treatment of arterial and venous disease

Dr Andrew Kelion
Harefield Hospital,
Royal Brompton and Harefield NHS Trust,
Middlesex, UK
Chapter 7: Perioperative management of ischaemic heart disease

Dr Mark Stoneham
Nuffield Department of Anaesthesia,
John Radcliffe Hospital, Oxford
Chapter 8: Anaesthesia for vascular surgery

Symbols and abbreviations

↓	decreased
↑	increased
⚠	warning
AAA	abdominal aortic aneurysm
ABPI	ankle brachial pressure index
ABF	aortobifemoral
AF	atrial fibrillation
AP	anteroposterior
APTT	activated partial thromboplastin time
ARDS	acute respiratory distress syndrome
ASG	aortic stent graft
AVP	ambulatory venous pressure
ASIS	anterior superior iliac spine
AT	anterior tibial (artery)
ATN	acute tubular necrosis
AV	arteriovenous
bd	twice a day
BP	blood pressure
CABG	coronary artery bypass graft
CCA	common carotid artery
CCF	congestive cardiac failure
CEA	carotid endarterectomy
CFA	common femoral artery
CIA	common iliac artery
COPD	chronic obstructive pulmonary disease
CRP	C reactive protein
CSF	cerebrospinal fluid
CT	computerized tomography
CTA	computerized tomography arteriogram
CVA	cardiovascular accident
CVI	chronic venous insufficiency
CVP	central venous pressure
CXR	chest X-ray
DSMO	dimethylsulphoxide
DVT	deep vein thrombosis
ECA	external carotid artery
ECG	electrocardiogram

EEG	electroencephalogram
EIA	external iliac artery
EPO	erythropoietin
ePTFE	expanded polytetrafluorethylene
ESR	erythrocyte sedimentation rate
ETCO$_2$	end-tidal carbon dioxide
ETT	endotracheal tube
EVLT	endovenous laser therapy
FFP	fresh frozen plasma
GA	general anaesthetic
GFR	glomerular filtration rate
GM-CSF	granulocyte–macrophage colony-stimulating factor
GSV	greater saphenous vein
GTN	glyceryl trinitrate
Hb	haemoglobin
HDL	high density lipoprotein
HDU	high dependency unit
HIT	heparin-induced thrombocytopaenia
ICA	internal carotid artery
IPPV	intermittent positive pressure ventilation
ICU	intensive care unit
IL-11	interleukin-11
INR	international normalized ratio
ITU	intensive therapy unit
IU	international units
iv	intravenous
IVC	inferior vena cava
IVI	intravenous infusion
JVP	jugular venous pressure
LA	local anaesthetic
LDL	low density lipoprotein
LMA	laryngeal mask airway
LMWH	low molecular weight heparin
LSV	lesser saphenous vein
LV	left ventricle
MI	myocardial infarction
MRA	magnetic resonance arteriography
MRI	magnetic resonance imaging
MRV	magnetic resonance venography
MPS	myocardial perfusion scintigraphy

MRSA	methicillin-resistant *Staphylococcus aureus*
NG	nasogastric
NIDDM	non-insulin dependent diabetes mellitus
NSAID	nonsteroidal anti-inflammatory drug
OCP	oral contraceptive pill
od	once a day
PA	pulmonary artery
PAD	peripheral arterial disease
PAOD	peripheral arterial occlusive disease
PCA	patient-controlled analgesia
PCI	percutaneous coronary intervention
PDS	polydioxanone
PE	pulmonary embolus
PICC	peripherally introduced central catheter
po	orally, by mouth
POBA	plain old balloon angioplasty
PSV	peak systolic velocity
PT	posterior tibial (artery) or prothrombin time
PTA	percutaneous transluminal angioplasty
PTFE	polytetrafluoroethylene
PSV	peak systolic velocity
qds	4 times a day
RCT	randomized controlled trial
RFA	radiofrequency ablation
rHuEPO	recombinant human erythropoietin
RT	refilling time
rt-PA	recombinant tissue plasminogen activator
sc	subcutaneous
SFA	superficial femoral artery
SFJ	sapheno-femoral junction
SMA	superior mesenteric artery
SPECT	single-photon emission computerized tomography
SPJ	sapheno-popliteal junction
SpO_2	oxygen saturation measured by pulse oximetry
STD	sodium tetradecyl sulphate
STIR	short tau inversion recovery (MRI sequence)
SVC	superior vena cava
SVR	systemic vascular resistance
tds	three times a day
TEG	thromboelastography

TFA	transfemoral angiogram
TIA	transient ischaemic attack
tPA	tissue plasminogen activator
TPN	total parenteral nutrition
U & E	urea and electrolytes
VDU	visual display unit
WCC	white blood cell count

Arterial and venous disease

Arterial disease: atherosclerosis

Atherosclerosis literally means 'hardening gruel' (*athere* (Gk) = gruel or porridge) and describes the development of the characteristic plaque or atheroma that builds up under the arterial endothelium over time. Atherosclerosis is generally asymptomatic until it causes significant narrowing of an artery (> 70%) or ruptures into the lumen generating thrombus and/or thromboemboli. It accounts for 40% of UK deaths.

Pathological stages (Fig. 1.1)
- Subintimal fatty streak.
- Inflammatory process in media.
- Build-up of fatty macrophages (foam cells).
- Progressive narrowing of arteries.
- Plaque rupture or ulceration.
- Thrombosis with occlusion or thromboembolism.

Risk factors

Atherosclerosis is an inflammatory condition and its progression and tendency for complications are strongly influenced by:
- smoking;
- hypertension;
- renal disease;
- diabetes;
- hypercholesterolaemia;
- family history.

Characteristics of atherosclerosis
- Systemic disease.
- Predilection for:
  - coronary arteries;
  - carotid arteries;
  - lower limb arteries;
  - visceral/renal arteries.
- Disease progression affected by risk factor control.

Size of the problem
- Heart disease and ischaemic stroke constitute the leading causes of death in the developed countries of the world and cause nearly a third of all deaths annually in North America and Europe.
- The annual number of myocardial infarctions in the USA and the EU is 2.1 million, and the number of ischaemic strokes is 1.75 million.
- A quarter of men and one-fifth of women will suffer a stroke between the ages of 45 and 85 years.
- Peripheral vascular disease is clinically manifest as intermittent claudication in almost 7% of the population aged 50–75 years.
- Different manifestations of atherosclerotic disease commonly coexist in the same patient (Fig. 1.2).

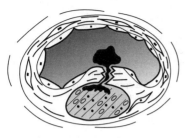

Fig. 1.1 Atheromatous plaque in artery.

Prevalence of vascular disease in a population 62 years of age and over

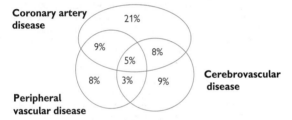

Fig. 1.2 Coexistence of coronary, cerebral, and peripheral vascular disease.

Coronary artery disease

Coronary atherosclerosis may present with angina or infarction but significant cardiac ischaemia sometimes remains asymptomatic. It can be assumed that patients presenting with carotid or peripheral arterial atherosclerotic disease have some degree of coronary disease. This is important in planning intervention but also forms the premise for stringent risk factor control. Correctable coronary artery disease may be a treatment priority in patients presenting with other clinical manifestations of atherosclerosis.

Carotid artery disease

Atherosclerosis of the carotid arteries shows a remarkable predilection for the origins of the internal and external carotid arteries, a fact that makes it amenable to carotid endarterectomy. Haemodynamic factors of shear and turbulence patterns at the bifurcation may be implicated in pathogenesis.

The majority of symptomatic disease is thought to be related to thromboembolic events resulting from plaque ulceration, platelet aggregation, and thrombosis. Stroke may also result from hypoperfusion caused by a significant narrowing, particularly in the context of hypotension, labile blood pressure, or contralateral internal/common carotid occlusion.

Peripheral arterial occlusive disease (PAOD)

Atherosclerotic disease particularly affects the aorto-iliac arteries, femoral arteries, popliteal and distal vessels. The disease is rarely isolated to one segment and is also usually bilateral. Significant stenosis may present with claudication. Claudication is most common in the calf with stenosis at any level; thigh or buttock claudication results from aorto-iliac disease. Claudication may remain stable (approximately 1/3), improve (approximately 1/3), or progress with symptoms coming after shorter distances (approximately 1/3).

Extreme progression of disease will result in threatened limb viability or critical ischaemia in less than 5% of claudicants. This is heralded clinically by the onset of rest pain in the forefoot or tissue loss presenting as ulceration, necrosis, or gangrene in the extremity. Critical ischaemia represents advanced atherosclerotic disease and signifies multiple level disease. Revascularization is required to maintain limb viability. This may involve angioplasty, stenting, surgical bypass, or any combination of these.

Renovascular disease Significant stenosis of the renal arteries can produce hypertension and renal failure. As with coronary artery disease this may require treatment before any other vascular intervention.

Visceral artery disease Although frequently affected by atherosclerosis, visceral artery ischaemia is rarely symptomatic because of the rich arterial collateral supply around the gut. Mesenteric ischaemia can result from coexistent coeliac axis and superior mesenteric artery disease.

Thromboembolic arterial disease

- An embolus is any substance that is transported from one part of the circulation to another.
- Thromboemboli most commonly arise in the heart in association with atrial fibrillation or subendocardial infarction, sometimes from thrombus on atherosclerotic plaques or aneurysms. They can lodge anywhere downstream in the arterial circulation, most frequently at bifurcations (Fig. 1.3).
- When a major vessel is occluded by embolus acute symptoms will arise in the area supplied by the occluded arteries.
- Thromboembolism is often associated with underlying systemic morbidity or procoagulant states and can be associated with a high mortality.
- Acute lower limb ischaemia is the most common presentation but upper limb ischaemia, mesenteric ischaemia, and brain ischaemia can also occur.
- Management is directed at treating the ischaemia by restoring perfusion through an open or endoluminal approach using mechanical or thrombolytic means, followed by anticoagulation and possibly definitive treatment of the embolic source.

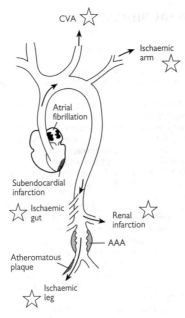

Fig. 1.3 Emboli in the arterial circulation.

Aneurysmal disease

See Fig. 1.4.

- An aneurysm is a permanent localized dilatation of an artery to more than 1.5 times its normal diameter.
- Aneurysms can be saccular or fusiform in shape.
- True aneurysms represent expansion of the arterial wall and include the following.
  - 'Atherosclerotic' aneurysm. The vast majority are associated with, but not necessarily caused by, atherosclerosis, usually fusiform, and the wall shows degenerative changes with loss of normal architecture and abnormalities of the connective tissue with defects in collagen and elastin content.
  - Mycotic aneurysms due to arterial wall infection, often saccular. Staphylococcal and salmonella organisms are most often implicated but they can be associated with fungal infection (hence the term mycotic).
  - Dissecting aneurysms due to longitudinal disruption of arterial wall integrity by a dissecting channel of parallel blood flow arising from the main lumen (see later in this section).
- False aneurysms are associated with penetrating trauma to the artery (needle, knife blade, bone spike, etc.) or breakdown of an arterial anastomosis, which results in escape of blood outside the artery. A fibrotic wall grows around the extravasated blood, which still maintains continuity with the main bloodstream and forms a saccular aneurysm lacking the normal three arterial layers of a 'true' aneurysm.
- Thrombus accumulates in the dilated portion of the artery.
- Aneurysms are generally asymptomatic until they rupture or cause ischaemia by thrombosis or thromboembolism.
- Aneurysms have been described throughout the arterial tree, but outside the cranium are most found most commonly in:
  - aorta;
  - popliteal arteries;
  - iliac arteries;
  - common femoral arteries;
  - visceral arteries;
  - renal arteries;
  - carotid arteries.

Abdominal aortic aneurysm

- Affects 5% of men over 60.
- Arises below the renal arteries in 95% of cases.
- Generally asymptomatic until rupture (most commonly) or lower limb ischaemia due to distal embolization. Usually diagnosed incidentally.

Risk factors for aortic aneurysm

- Male sex.
- Positive family history.
- Smoking.
- Hypertension.

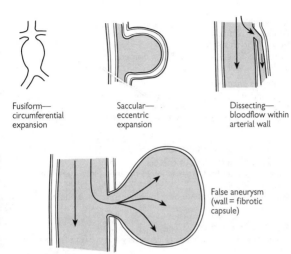

Fusiform—
circumferential
expansion

Saccular—
eccentric
expansion

Dissecting—
bloodflow within
arterial wall

False aneurysm
(wall = fibrotic
capsule)

Fig. 1.4 Types of aneurysms.

Risk of rupture
This is directly related to aneurysm size:
- rare in aneurysms < 4cm diameter;
- increases to 5% per annum at 5.5cm diameter;
- rises exponentially thereafter.

Inflammatory aneurysm
This accounts for up to 10% of cases. There is a generalized inflammation of the arterial wall, which may involve peri-aortic tissue, causing pain and occasionally ureteric obstruction. Open repair of these cases is technically difficult.

Thoraco-abdominal aneurysms
- Arise from the aortic arch or descending aorta.
- Present a greater challenge than infrarenal aneurysms in terms of risk of intervention.
- Endovascular techniques are now the most common mode of treatment.

Iliac artery aneurysms
- Arise in the common or internal iliac artery and are usually associated with aortic aneurysm.
- May be complicated by thrombosis or rupture.
- Are excluded during aortic aneurysm repair. When they occur in isolation, elective repair or exclusion is advocated to prevent rupture at a size of 4cm or greater.
- Can often be treated endovascularly.

Popliteal aneurysms
- Account for 80% of peripheral artery aneurysms beyond the aorta.
- Are associated with aortic aneurysm in 30% of cases. 50% are bilateral.
- Most common complication is leg ischaemia due to thrombotic occlusion or thromboembolism. Limb ischaemia associated with popliteal aneurysm carries a high incidence of limb loss.
- Rarely cause compression symptoms, deep venous thrombosis, or rupture.

Common femoral artery aneurysm
- In its true form is less common than false aneurysm or post-anastomotic aneurysm at the same site.
- 25% of true aneurysms are associated with an aortic aneurysm.

Visceral artery aneurysms
- Rare but occur most often in the hepatic or splenic arteries.
- Splenic artery aneurysm is associated with pregnancy.
- Rupture is a recognized complication with a high mortality. Repair (often endovascular) is advocated for incidentally discovered aneurysm of 2cm diameter or more.

Carotid artery aneurysm
- Rare.

- Exclusion is recommended to prevent rupture and can be accomplished with open or endovascular techniques.
- Anastamotic aneurysm following previous closure or patch of carotid endarterectomy should be treated similarly.

Dissecting aneurysms

- Dissection occurs spontaneously most often in the thoracic aorta. Type A arises from the arch; type B from below the left subclavian artery.
- Arises when a false lumen develops from blood tracking into the arterial wall through an intimal tear.
- Classical presentation is acute onset of severe chest pain radiating through to the back between the scapulae, and associated with hypertension.
- May be complicated by upper limb, cerebral, visceral, renal, or lower limb ischaemia.
- Diagnosis is confirmed on CT angiography.
- Treatment.
  - Type A cases usually require aortic arch and sometimes aortic valve replacement.
  - Type B cases with no evidence of significant ischaemia or pending rupture can be treated medically with analgesia and blood pressure control.
  - Endovascular covered stents are the treatment of choice for cases complicated by ischaemia (usually lower limb, renal, or visceral), a contained aortic rupture, early aortic expansion after presentation, or unrelenting pain.
  - Open surgery with fenestration of the dissection and circumferential tacking of intima to artery wall below this point may be required if stenting proves impossible.
- Carotid dissection may present with stroke. Treatment is generally conservative.

Raynaud's phenomenon

- Vasospastic disorder that presents as painful discolouration of the digits on exposure to cold and certain other stimuli.
- High female preponderance.
- May be associated with connective tissue disorders, Buerger's disease, cervical rib, use of vibrating tools ('vibration white finger').
- Neurogenic mechanisms and inflammatory changes in the vessel wall are thought to be important.

Large vessel arteritis

Group of disorders involving arterial inflammation that present as peripheral ischaemia, with necrosis of soft tissues of the extremities in association with systemic symptoms of malaise. Although clinical picture is often of stenotic disease, arterial wall 'softening' from inflammation may occasionally produce aneurysms. Diagnosis is based on clinical picture and distribution of disease. Inflammatory markers may be raised. A confirmatory histological diagnosis is not always obtained.

Takayasu's disease

- Causes stenosis of aortic branches (including coronary arteries) and other major arteries (also known as the 'pulseless disease').
- Commonest in women in 2nd and 3rd decades.
- Initial acute inflammation of media and adventitia followed by scarring and thickening of intima, leading to stenosis.
- Occasionally causes aneurysms of aorta.
- Main treatment is immunosuppression in acute inflammatory stage. Occasionally balloon angioplasty or surgery is required in later stages.

Buerger's disease

- Inflammation of medium-sized arteries and veins.
- Affects male smokers, particularly of eastern Mediterranean, Middle Eastern, and Asian origin.
- Closely related to cigarette smoking.
- Transmural inflammation associated with luminal thrombus and macrophages.
- Causes occlusion of forearm arteries in upper limb and crural vessels in lower limbs leading to claudication, rest pain, and tissue necrosis.
- Characteristic 'corkscrew' collaterals sometimes seen on angiography.
- Treatment is smoking cessation. Prostacyclin infusion occasionally helps.

Giant cell (temporal) arteritis

- Affects mainly women, usually > 50 years old.
- Prodromal 'flu-like' illness over 2–3 weeks followed by limb girdle muscle pain; tender arteries, especially temporal, subclavian, axillary, brachial, and superficial femoral; and amaurosis fugax or permanent

blindness. Occasionally limb claudication; rarely ischaemic lesions peripherally. Symptoms develop over several months.
- ESR usually > 80; mild normochromic anaemia.
- Responds to steroids, which reverse arterial stenosis but not occlusion.

Rheumatoid vasculitis

- Acute vasculitis in association with rheumatoid arthritis.
- Affects small- to medium-sized arteries potentially anywhere except lung.
- Can produce 'punched out' ulcers on shins and digital gangrene.
- Responds to steroids or other immunosuppression.

Polyarteritis nodosa

- Affects medium-sized arteries.
- May be associated with aneurysmal dilatation.
- Causes ischaemia in gut, kidneys, and brain most commonly.
- Can cause purpura or gangrenous patches in the skin when small aneurysms may be felt as nodules associated with arteries.
- Association with hepatitis B.

Other arterial disorders

Diabetic vascular disease A combination of large vessel atherosclerotic disease (which is 2–3 times commoner in the diabetic population) and disruption of microcirculatory control.

Fibromuscular dysplasia

- Disease of the arterial media that causes stenosis.
- Affects young women in 90% of cases and occurs in the absence of atherosclerotic risk factors.
- Affects mainly the renal and carotid arteries.
- May give a beaded appearance on angiography.
- Angioplasty is the treatment of choice.

Cystic adventitial disease

- Disease of adventitia.
- Affects the popliteal artery most commonly.
- May cause claudication in young patients.
- Well demonstrated on duplex.
- Usually treated surgically by drainage of cyst with vein interposition graft only required if popliteal artery thrombosed.

Carotid body tumour

- Uncommon tumour of the carotid body.
- Usually slow-growing and benign.
- Member of paraganglioma tumour family (includes phaeochromocytoma) but rarely secretes catecholamines.
- Presents as a swelling in the neck, which may be tender.
- May cause problems with cranial nerves (IX, X, XI, XII) due to pressure as it grows.
- Duplex is useful as an initial investigation and shows classically splaying of the internal and external carotids. MRI or CT confirms the diagnosis and differentiates from vagal body tumours; also useful in demonstrating upper extent of tumour if not seen clearly on duplex.
- Resection is indicated in younger patients; preoperative embolization may be helpful in reducing vascularity and shrinking if large. Radiotherapy may shrink (but not cure) tumour and is indicated in elderly patient with large/symptomatic tumour.

Venous disease: introduction

The great majority of venous disease is accounted for by three interrelated conditions:
- varicose veins;
- deep venous thrombosis;
- chronic venous insufficiency.

Normal venous physiology

- Venous return is achieved through the complex arrangement of arterial inflow, negative pressure of respiration, unidirectional valves, and muscle pumps (Fig. 1.5).
- The upright position presents the greatest physiological challenge to lower limb venous return against gravity.
- Normally, activation of the muscular 'pump' can deal readily with venous return from the lower limb, but inadequacy of the pump or loss of valve function can lead to venous pooling and complications such as varicosities, thrombophlebitis, skin changes, and ulceration.

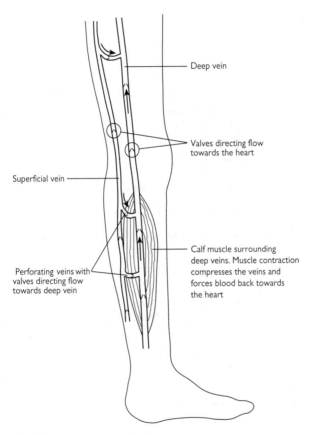

Fig. 1.5 Normal venous return from the leg.

Varicose veins

- Dilated tortuous superficial veins that occur almost exclusively in the lower limb.
- Affect at least 40% of the Western population to some degree.
- Vast majority are 'primary' (see below) but occasionally secondary to DVT or pelvic venous obstruction by tumour or by deep venous incompetence.
- Histology shows abnormal architecture with reduction in normal elastin and altered collagen matrix.
- Varicosities are generally classified as:
  - truncal varicosities;
  - reticular varicosities or tributaries;
  - hyphenweb, spider veins, thread veins, or telangiectases.

Aetiology of primary varicose veins

- Cause is unknown but probably arise as part of an inflammatory process that may be associated with long periods of venous hypertension.
- Strongly associated with valvular incompetence but whether this results from the same inflammatory process or necessarily precedes the development of varicosities is not known.
- Truncal incompetence will further accelerate the varicose process by promoting venous distension and reducing venous return.
- Greater saphenous vein (GSV) is incompetent in at least 80% people with varicose veins; lesser saphenous vein (LSV) in about 15%.
- Direct role of incompetent perforators in the development of varicosities is not universally agreed but they undoubtedly contribute to calf pump insufficiency.

Complications of varicose veins

- **Haemorrhage**. Most likely to occur from intradermal varices, which are very superficial and subject to trauma. Can be profuse.
- **Thrombophlebitis**. Painful inflammation of the varicose vein with associated thrombosis of the vein. Thrombosis of the vein can be extensive and it spreads to include DVT in approximately 10% of cases.

Chronic venous insufficiency

- Associated with superficial and/or deep venous disease.
- Produces skin changes that correlate with failure of the calf pump to reduce ambulatory venous pressure (see Chapter 4, Fig. 4.3, p. 63) and are thought to result from prolonged distension of veins with stagnant blood.
- Skin changes of chronic venous insufficiency:
  - oedema;
  - pigmentation;
  - eczema;
  - lipodermatosclerosis;
  - ulceration.
- Skin changes are usually, but not always, associated with varicose veins.
- Classified according to the CEAP system (see box and Table 1.1).

CEAP system

C   Clinical signs (graded 0–6), supplemented by (s) for symptomatic and (a) for asymptomatic presentation

E   (A)etiological classification (congenital, primary, secondary)

A   Anatomical distribution (superficial, deep, or perforator, alone or in combination)

P   Pathophysiological dysfunction (reflux or obstruction, alone or in combination)

Table 1.1 CEAP clinical classification of chronic venous disease*

Class	Clinical signs
0	No visible or palpable signs of venous disease
1	Telangiectases, reticular veins, malleolar flare
2	Varicose veins
3	Oedema without skin changes
4	Skin changes ascribed to venous disease (pigmentation, venous eczema, lipodermatosclerosis)
5	Skin changes (as defined above) in conjunction with healed ulceration
6	Skin changes (as defined above) in conjunction with active ulceration

* See box on facing page for explanation of 'CEAP'.

Deep venous thrombosis (DVT)

- Usually originates in the calf (soleal) veins.
- Starts with platelet–endothelial (or leucocyte–endothelial) activation of the thrombotic cascade usually in a valve sinus; further deposition of platelets and fibrin forms an adherent thrombus. Continued activation of the clotting system will result in thrombus propagation.
- Propagated thrombus is less adherent and at risk of breaking off and embolizing.

Clinical consequences of DVT

- Painful leg swelling.
- Pulmonary embolism (PE).
- Chronic venous insufficiency (post-phlebitic limb).
- More rarely:
  - paradoxical embolus—in association with a patent foramen ovale;
  - phlegmasia caerulea dolens—in association with a massive ilio-femoral DVT.

Risk factors for DVT

- Past history of DVT/PE.
- Increasing age.
- Immobility.
- Malignancy.
- Surgery or other trauma.
- Cardiac failure, stroke, and MI.
- Oral contraceptive pill (OCP).
- Thrombophilia (see p. 158).

Pulmonary embolism (PE)

- Occurs when propagated clot breaks off and embolizes through the right heart to occlude the pulmonary arteries.
- Fatal PE can occur in up to 10% of patients with DVT with the risks being highest in those with proximal extension of the DVT. Those patients with thrombus confined to the calf veins (i.e. below the popliteal vein) are at low risk of PE.
- PE classically presents with sudden onset of dyspnoea, chest pain, cough, and haemoptysis, with associated tachycardia, tachypnoea, and distress. However, the symptoms may be protean.
- Paradoxical embolism can occur in the presence of a patent foramen ovale (present in 20% of normal people), which allows the embolus to enter the left side of the heart and travel in the arterial circulation, lodging at any site of narrowing, usually in the lower limb where it may present as acute limb ischaemia.

Phlegmasia caerulea dolens

- An uncommon complication of DVT.
- Occurs with ilio-femoral DVT when major obstruction of venous return impedes capillary flow with a subsequent reduction in arterial inflow.
- Presents with massively swollen, blue–purple discolouration of the limb and ischaemia followed by necrosis of the toes.
- Often seen in association with severe illness such as disseminated malignancy where there is a poor prognosis.
- Treatment is limb elevation and anticoagulation. Catheter-directed thrombolysis should also be considered in those with less co-morbidity.

Post-phlebitic limb

- DVT normally resolves over a period of weeks to months leaving patent but often incompetent deep veins. Chronically obstructed deep veins will give similar results.
- Reflux or obstruction in the deep veins promotes venous pooling and stasis with oedema and inflammation, development of skin changes, and varicosities.
- Ultimately, the classic post-phlebitic limb, with oedema, varicose veins, haemosiderin deposition, lipodermatosclerosis, and intractable ulceration, may develop.
- These changes may be prevented by prolonged use of compression stockings and limb elevation when possible.
- Superficial vein surgery is likely to be less effective in patients with underlying deep vein insufficiency.

Upper limb venous thrombosis

- Usually subclavian/axillary vein thrombosis (Paget–Schroetter syndrome).
- Less common than lower limb DVT and often associated with an underlying abnormality causing obstruction of the venous outflow:
  - subclavian vein stenosis;
  - sepsis (Lemierre's syndrome);
  - thoracic outlet (inlet) syndrome with compression from ribs or bands;
  - central venous catheterization;
  - thrombophilia;
  - effort syndrome (repetitive shoulder movements).
- The risk of progression to pulmonary embolism and post-phlebitic syndrome is low and full anticoagulation is less strongly indicated.

Uncommon venous disorders

Klippel–Trenaunay syndrome

- A congenital condition of the mesoderm in which there are gross widespread varicosities associated with port wine stains and bone and soft tissue hypertrophy producing limb overgrowth.
- Occurs with equal frequency in both sexes.
- Can affect one or both lower limbs.
- Non-operative management is indicated in most cases.

Arteriovenous fistulae

- Occasionally found with varicosities and skin ischaemia.
- Duplex useful for diagnosis.
- Rarely leads to high output heart failure.
- Management primarily endovascular if causing significant problems; otherwise leave alone.

Leiomyomatosis/leiomyosarcoma

- Rare extension of uterine fibroma/sarcoma into the venous system.
- Spreads to involve the IVC and right heart, and presents with heart failure.
- Often mistakenly diagnosed as DVT.
- Treatment is resection.

Arterial history and examination

Peripheral arterial history: introduction

As with many areas of medicine, the history is the most important means of determining the following:

- Is this problem due to arterial disease (occlusive or aneurysmal)?
- How severe is any ischaemia (claudication/rest pain/tissue loss)?

The following sections cover areas to concentrate on in the vascular patient.

Presenting symptoms

Pain

Site

- Muscle (commonly calf, sometimes thigh or buttock, occasionally forearm) suggests claudication. Buttock claudication is caused by aorto-iliac disease but this is the only circumstance in which site of pain reveals level of arterial obstruction; aorto-iliac disease is more commonly associated with calf claudication.
- Forefoot or finger tips (periphery of circulation) suggests ischaemic rest pain.

Nature

- Cramping/tightness/gripping sensation suggest claudication.
- Constant/gnawing ache (often severe) is typical of rest pain.

Precipitating factors

- Claudication is only felt with exercise.
- Rest pain is exacerbated by elevation, e.g. going to bed.

Relieving factors

- Claudication pain disappears within a few minutes (< 5min) of stopping exercise. Leg claudication is relieved by standing still. Bending over or sitting down (see 'Spinal stenosis', p. 30) do not ease it any more quickly.
- Ischaemic rest pain is relieved by dependency.

Numbness/tingling If present, usually felt in the forefoot or finger tips.

Ulceration/gangrene Occur either in the forefoot/fingers or over pressure areas in the foot (including heel); occasionally over malleoli if fixed external/internal rotation of hip for any reason. Painful.

Erectile impotence A common problem in older men for a number of reasons but may be caused by aorto-iliac disease (in association with buttock claudication known as Leriche's syndrome).

Differential diagnosis

PAOD is common and often asymptomatic. The absence of pulses in elderly patients does not necessarily indicate that the problem is due to arterial disease. The most important differential information for making the diagnosis comes from the history, particularly when the patient is complaining of leg or foot pain.

Claudication

The patient who presents with leg pain on walking may have claudication but the following differential diagnoses are of common conditions in older people and need to be considered.

Osteoarthritis

- Most difficult when hip pain presents as thigh discomfort. Ankle pain is sometimes difficult to differentiate from calf pain. Knee pain is usually easy to distinguish from its site (anterior).
- Ask about time course of pain during the day and time to recovery after exercise. Claudication distance and recovery time are generally stable throughout the day, whereas osteoarthritic pain gets worse during the day and gradually takes longer to wear off.
- If at any stage the pain takes more than 5 minutes to wear off after exercise it is **not** claudication.

Sciatica

- Usually a sharp shooting pain rather than cramping or tightness.
- Ask if it comes on when leaning forward to get out of a chair or bending over.
- Claudication pain only occurs in association with walking or running.

Spinal stenosis

- An uncommon condition, but found more often in the vascular clinic because of the difficulty in differentiating from vascular claudication (hence its alternative name of 'neurogenic claudication').
- Patient complains of calf pain on walking, which is relieved fairly quickly by rest.
- Classically patient has to flex the spine by bending over or sitting to relieve the discomfort. It does not get better (or at least does so only slowly) if patient remains upright.
- Ask if the same pain ever occurs when standing, especially at the sink when the spine tends to be more extended. **If so it cannot be vascular claudication**. Ask what they have to do to relieve the pain.

Ischaemic rest pain

Foot pain is commonly caused by the following conditions in the older patient.

- **Osteoarthritis of the foot**. Usually deteriorates during the day. Unlike ischaemic rest pain, it is relieved by elevating (taking weight off) the foot.

- **Gout** may be difficult to differentiate from secondary infection in an ischaemic foot (swelling obscures foot pulses) but pain is often relieved by elevation (unlike ischaemic rest pain).
- **Peripheral neuropathy** is a common differential in diabetic patients.
  - Usually described as a burning or shooting pain affecting most of the foot rather than a constant pain affecting the forefoot.
  - Sometimes worse in bed but usually does not have clear cut exacerbation with elevation.

Assessing severity of the problem

- Ischaemic rest pain type symptoms or ulceration/gangrene indicate greater severity of disease than claudication symptoms alone.
- Patient's estimate of distance to onset of claudication and maximum walking distance (the level of disability) are a measure of disease severity: useful as a baseline for comparison over time or post-intervention.
- Patient's description of limitations imposed by claudication, e.g. can no longer walk the dog or get to the shops (the level of handicap), is a good guide as to whether intervention is justified for claudication.

Modifiable risk factors and associated disease

Modifiable risk factors

These need to be recorded so that any options for modifying them and reducing risk of disease progression can be explored. They are, in order of importance:

- smoking (record 'pack years' and time since stopping);
- diabetes;
- hypertension;
- dyslipidaemia;
- family history of early onset arterial disease (< 60y)—usually due to raised cholesterol but occasionally other factors important, e.g. hyperhomocysteinaemia.

Associated disease

Several diseases are commonly associated with peripheral arterial disease because they are also either caused by atherosclerosis or by smoking. They are important for the following reasons.

- They may restrict what intervention can be performed without undue risk to the patient's life.
- They may suggest that patient survival (as opposed to limb survival) demands more urgent intervention elsewhere, e.g. coronary angiography for severe coexistent angina.
- They may limit exercise to the extent that any intervention for claudication would be of limited benefit.

The important diseases to ask about are:

- coronary artery disease. Ask about chest pain, angina, heart attack.
- cerebrovascular disease. Ask about stroke and TIA.
- renal artery disease. Common association but difficult to elicit on history unless already diagnosed. Causes hypertension and renal failure. The former is a common finding in PAD but usually 'essential' rather than secondary to renal artery stenosis.
- chronic obstructive pulmonary disease (COPD). Ask about shortness of breath, cough, wheezing, etc.

Medication

One would hope that any patient referred with PAOD is already on a platelet inhibitor. Sadly, this is often not the case. The following drugs are of particular importance:

- antiplatelet agents: aspirin, clopidogrel, dipyridamole;
- cholesterol lowering agents: statins, fibrates;
- warfarin: may need stopping prior to investigation or treatment;
- metformin: needs to be stopped before intravascular contrast investigations;
- β-blockers: may make claudication worse but provide beneficial perioperative cardiac protection.

Social history

Mobility, particularly on stairs, is likely to be restricted in these patients, so access to home (e.g. 6th floor apartment or groundfloor accommodation) is important to establish. Some may come to amputation so potential for wheelchair access is also important (ramps, door widths, toilet, and washing facilities on the same level as rest of accommodation, etc.). Most of these latter details will be clarified by a home visit by an occupational therapist or similarly qualified individual but a rough idea of potential problems at the outset can allow the appropriate agencies to be alerted early and possibly avoid unduly delayed discharge from hospital. Social support available to the patient in the form of relatives or friends should also be noted because this may dictate how well they can manage in the community.

Examination for PAOD: systemic assessment

It is tempting to concentrate on the offending limb, having heard so much about it in the history. Avoid this pitfall. You must assess the whole patient first as systemic factors may contribute significantly to the development of limb symptoms.

Systemic assessment involves a routine physical examination of all systems but should concentrate particularly on the following two areas.

Quality of circulation

- Evidence of 'forward failure': pulse volume (and note whether in atrial fibrillation); temperature and colour of hands; blood pressure.
- Evidence of 'backward failure': unable to lie flat; raised JVP; crepitations in basal lung fields; ankle oedema. Beware: this last sign can also be caused by sleeping in a chair because of rest pain.

Quality of circulating blood

- Evidence of anaemia: check conjunctiva.
- Evidence of polycythaemia (e.g. $2°$ to smoking): look for plethoric complexion.
- Evidence of hypoxia (e.g. $2°$ to COPD): look for central cyanosis.
- Evidence of hypercholesterolaemia: check for xanthelasma, corneal arcus (if < 60).

Local assessment

There are three questions to be asked when examining the affected limb and comparison should be made with the contralateral limb where possible.

1. Is there evidence of arterial obstruction or aneurysmal dilatation?

This is determined by palpation of pulses, with the patient lying as flat as possible (Table 2.1).

Aorta

- Palpate the epigastrium.
- Most aortas will be impalpable but it is important to check for an abdominal aortic aneurysm (AAA).
- Detection of midline pulsation with a finger in the umbilicus suggests an AAA but needs ultrasound confirmation (the normal aortic bifurcation lies just above the umbilicus but is pushed distally by aneurysmal elongation of the aorta).

Femoral pulses

- If difficult to find, check bony landmarks. Find them either:
    - 2/3 down a line from the anterior superior iliac spine (ASIS) to the pubic tubercle (felt by sweeping finger up from groin rather than trying to push down through suprapubic fat pad); or
    - halfway between ASIS and pubic symphysis (midline).
- If still not palpable then externally rotate the hip to push the artery forward with the femoral head.
- Femoral pulses may be aneurysmal, normal, reduced, or absent. Apparently normal pulses may mask significant upstream disease so always listen for a femoral bruit as well.

Popliteal pulses

These are often difficult to feel but don't be tempted to miss them out as they may be aneurysmal. Feel just lateral to the midline in the popliteal fossa with the leg either straight and relaxed, or flexed (get used to whichever of these methods seems to suit you best).

Pedal pulses

Dorsalis pedis: on dorsum of foot between tendons of extensor hallucis longus and tibialis anterior, in 1st metatarsal space. Posterior tibial: approximately 1cm posterior to medial malleolus.

Although there is often diffuse atherosclerosis affecting limb blood supply, it is common for there to be one or two sites of haemodynamically significant disease that can be targeted for intervention. Palpation of pulses will allow you to find the most proximal level of significant disease but will not inform you of the distal extent.

Table 2.1 The commonest sites of significant disease, their prevalence in the PAOD population, and the resultant findings on pulse palpation

Disease site	Prevalence	Findings
Superficial femoral artery	70%	Femoral but no distal pulses
Aorto-iliac disease	20%	Reduced, absent, or normal femoral pulse with a bruit. Usually no distal pulses
Infrapopliteal disease*	10%	Femoral & popliteal pulses only

* Common in diabetic and very elderly patients.

2. How severe is the ischaemia?

You will already have some idea of this from the patient's symptoms. Look for the following on examination with the patient lying down, comparing the two feet where appropriate (Fig. 2.1).

- Ulcers (usually 'punched out' in profile) or gangrene affecting the forefoot (look between the toes) or pressure areas (especially medial and lateral aspects, respectively, of 1st and 5th metatarso-phalangeal joints and back of heel).
- Colour of foot.
  - Dusky red indicates chronic ischaemia.
  - Pallor suggests acute ischaemia.
- Temperature of foot. Feel with palmar aspect of whole hand to get a global assessment.
- Capillary refill. Press gently over side or nail of 1st toe; then release and note speed with which pallor disappears. Usually < 3sec so record as 'normal', 'delayed', or 'very delayed' but don't go for spurious accuracy with terms such as '30sec capillary refill' when you haven't used a stopwatch.
- Buerger's test.
  - Stand at end of bed and lift both feet to about 45°; look for pallor of toes.
  - Replace feet on the bed and help the patient to sit up and swing their feet over the side of the bed. Look for redness of the forefoot greater than that with the legs horizontal.
  - This last step may take some time if there is severe arterial disease that slows blood flow into the foot to make it red.
  - Guttering of the foot veins in the early stage of foot dependency will give you a clue that ischaemia is severe.
  - Elevation pallor and dependent rubor indicate tissue ischaemia at rest.
- Fixed tissue staining. While lifting the feet during Buerger's test look for small patches of purplish discoloration in the toes or back of the heel suggesting capillary leak into the tissues due to severe ischaemia.

3. Is there infection?

This is a commoner problem in the patient with rest pain or tissue loss than in those with claudication. In diabetic patients it can quickly spread to cause widespread tissue necrosis in the foot or systemic sepsis. It is important to recognize the presence and extent of infection at an early stage. Look for:

- a red flare in the foot with the leg horizontal;
- a red flare extending up the leg indicating lymphatic tracking;
- a red flare tracking along a tendon indicating tendon sheath infection;
- crepitus in the subcutaneous tissue (especially in diabetic patients) indicating gas gangrene and the need for urgent amputation;
- fluctuation in the subcutaneous tissues suggesting abscess formation;
- a sinus with discharging pus suggesting deep infection;
- exposed bone in an ulcer base, which will inevitably be infected;
- a swollen red 'sausage' toe indicating osteomyelitis.

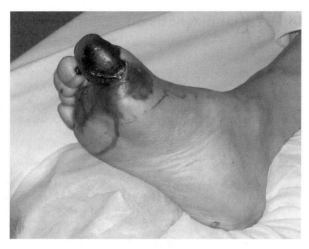

Fig. 2.1 The ischaemic foot.

Differential diagnosis on examination

Some areas of differential diagnosis have to wait until examination.

Gangrene

Gangrene is always due to impaired blood flow, but the problem may be in the large arteries (usually due to atherosclerosis or emboli), the medium-sized arteries (e.g. Buerger's disease, emboli), or the smallest arteries/arterioles (vasculitis, thrombosis, emboli). The differential diagnosis has to be based on an assessment of pulses and determination of likely precipitants (e.g. atrial fibrillation, heavy smoker, cold exposure).

Ulceration

Common alternative causes of ulceration in this population are as follows.
- Venous.
  - Almost always starts above the malleoli (usually on the medial side) but may spread to involve the foot.
  - Profile tends to reveal a sloping edge rather than punched out profile of arterial ulcer.
  - Surrounded by skin changes of chronic venous insufficiency.
  - Ulcer usually uncomfortable rather than very painful (as in ischaemia).
- Neuropathic. Common differential problem in diabetic patients.
  - Like ischaemic ulcers, found over pressure areas in the foot.
  - Presence of normal sensation and ulcer pain in the foot excludes this diagnosis.
  - Unfortunately, ischaemia and neuropathy commonly coexist and ulcer may be due to both factors.
  - Significant ischaemia prevents callus-build up around edge of ulcer so profile may allow you to differentiate.
- Malignant. Unusual in UK. Raised irregular edge and relative lack of pain should make you suspicious.

Venous history and examination

History: presenting symptoms

Venous disease may affect upper or lower limbs but more commonly the latter. The following symptoms are common to most venous disorders whether acute or chronic, affecting superficial or deep veins.

Pain

- Aching is the commonest symptom. It tends to accompany leg swelling and is felt generally in the lower leg towards the end of the day. It is relieved by putting the feet up.
- Acute episodes of pain persisting for more than a day are usually due to phlebitis, cellulitis, or possibly a DVT.
  - In phlebitis throbbing pain, sometimes quite severe, is felt along the line of a vein and is accompanied by redness in the same area.
  - Diffuse pain and redness, usually with generalized leg swelling, suggest cellulitis or a DVT.
- Calf muscle cramp disturbing sleep is found commonly in patients with venous disease.
- Restless leg syndrome is a chronic disorder in which there is a powerful urge to keep one or both legs moving to try and relieve a diffuse irritating leg discomfort. It often develops during the day so that the patient finds it impossible to sit still in the evening and sleep is disturbed. Restless leg syndrome can be caused by a number of disorders but is not uncommon in association with varicose veins. The discomfort is different from the ache when upright and is not relieved by elevation.

Swelling

Common in any venous disorder, this affects the foot and ankle and extends a variable distance up the leg. It is most pronounced in the evening and usually disappears (or, in the case of acute DVT, reduces) with overnight bed rest. Unless complicated by cellulitis, the swelling is painless. When asking patients about swelling be careful to differentiate between limb swelling and localized vein swelling (i.e. varicosities).

Non-venous causes of painless leg swelling

- Chronic lymphoedema is often slowly progressive over many years. It does not reduce with elevation overnight (unlike venous related oedema).
  - Congenital hypoplasia of the lymphatics often manifests in the 2nd or 3rd decade and usually affects both legs but one may be more advanced.
  - Post surgery that interrupts lymphatic drainage, e.g. inguinal lymph node clearance for malignancy, occasionally infrainguinal bypass graft.
  - Post pelvic or inguinal radiotherapy.
  - Infection causing obstruction or scarring of the lymphatics. Repeated episodes of non-specific calf cellulitis or specific infections such as filariasis.

- Congestive cardiac failure affects both legs equally and reduces with elevation. Usually associated with other symptoms such as orthopnoea and a history of cardiac disease.
- Hypoproteinaemia also affects both legs equally and reduces with elevation. Associated with low protein diet, gastrointestinal, liver, or renal disease.
- Prolonged inactive dependency, e.g. in a paralysed limb or in severe ischaemia when the patient sleeps in a chair or with the affected limb hanging over the side of the bed.

Distended superficial veins Varicose veins are a disorder well recognized by the general population and commonly self-diagnosed by the patient. They appear as a primary disorder or secondary to chronic deep venous disease. The appearance of dilated tortuous varicosities is profoundly disliked by many patients, particularly younger women. In the acute DVT superficial veins may become distended but this is rarely the most prominent symptom noticed by the patient.

Itching Although itching over a prominent varicosity or around the ankle is a symptom of venous disease, it can also be caused by dry skin. This is a common complaint, especially from women as they get older. Hot baths exacerbate the dryness.

Bleeding Most varicose veins are covered by a thick layer of skin and are unlikely to bleed with everyday trauma. A small group of patients develops protuberant venous blebs that erode through the skin and bleed spontaneously or with minor trauma such as drying the skin with a towel.

Skin discolouration

- Acute onset of redness, either localized to the line of a vein as in phlebitis or diffusely affecting the calf as in cellulitis or DVT, is not uncommon in venous disease.
- Some patients have insidious onset of discolouration, usually in the ankle region, due to chronic venous insufficiency. This includes brown staining, itchy red patches of eczema, paler patches (often painful) of atrophie blanche. Eczema may also appear over prominent varicosities higher in the leg. Find out if the patient has eczema elsewhere in the body: it may be unrelated to venous disease.

Ulceration

- This occurs in the ankle region and is usually associated with only mild to moderate discomfort, relieved by elevation. If the patient complains of marked pain, especially if dependency gives relief, suspect that there is an ischaemic component, usually due to coexistent PAOD.
- Many venous ulcers produce large volumes of exudate that seep through dressings on to the foot and smell, making the patient's life miserable. Find out how often the ulcer needs redressing.

Non-venous causes of lower leg ulceration

- Trauma—usually clear from the history.

- Vasculitis—usually multiple and in association with autoimmune disease such as rheumatoid arthritis.
- Pyoderma gangrenosum—starts as a tender red or blue skin nodule, which then breaks down centrally. May be associated with autoimmune disease.
- Buruli ulcer or other tropical infection.
- Malignancy, e.g. squamous cell carcinoma, basal cell carcinoma, malignant melanoma.

Having established that this is probably a venous problem then you must find out the likely cause.

History suggestive of acute DVT

Acute DVT is an important cause of venous disease, sometimes resulting in acute calf discomfort, swelling, redness, and superficial venous distension but often lacking some or all of these symptoms. Ilio-femoral DVT produces a more extreme form of presentation with swelling, discomfort, and venous engorgement throughout the limb. In the patient presenting with a possible DVT it is important to find out about possible contributory factors that would strengthen such a diagnosis. The patient should be asked specifically about:
- past venous thrombosis or pulmonary embolus;
- advanced age;
- malignancy;
- recent surgery (especially hip or knee joint replacement and pelvic surgery);
- leg trauma and/or immobilization (e.g. plaster cast);
- MI, CCF, stroke;
- air travel > 4h;
- use of oral contraceptive pill or hormone replacement therapy;
- inflammatory bowel disease.

History of past DVT

Many patients do not present at the time of DVT but months or years later with secondary varicose veins or skin changes. Certainly a past diagnosis of DVT should be asked about but may be negative. It is equally important to ask about likely precipitants of DVT in the past such as hip or knee replacement, pelvic surgery, leg fracture, or bad sprain, especially if immobilized in strapping or plaster cast.

History suggestive of chronic pelvic pathology

The vast majority of patients with venous symptoms have primary varicose veins or DVT-related pathology. A small number have a more sinister cause of their symptoms. Remember this, especially in the older patient who has recently developed venous symptoms. The iliac veins are easily compressed by a pelvic mass and may thrombose because of low flow, malignant infiltration, or spreading inflammation. Pelvic vein compression or thrombosis impairs venous drainage from the leg and results in leg swelling (often up to the groin—uncommon when the pathology is confined to the leg) and any of the other symptoms listed above as characteristic of venous disease. The commonest cause is an ovarian tumour.

- Find out if the patient still has her ovaries—in the past they were often removed with the uterus during hysterectomy for benign disease.
- Does the patient have urinary frequency, suggesting bladder compression or local inflammation?
- Is there frequency of stool evacuation suggesting pelvic inflammation?
- Has there been lower abdominal discomfort or weight loss?

Family history

- The commonest venous disorder, varicose veins, appear to run in families (although they are so common that, in the West at least, they appear to be a consequence of belonging to the human family, rather than any single family).
- There is some suggestion that the tendency to develop venous ulcers is hereditary.
- A family history of DVT or of repeated miscarriage is also important for it suggests a thrombophilic factor and an increased chance of DVT in the patient.

Examination

Ask the patient to stand and examine the legs looking for the following.

- Dilated tortuous (i.e. varicose) superficial veins indicating superficial incompetence. Decide:
  - are they are in the greater or lesser saphenous systems (Fig. 3.1)?
  - are they isolated minor varicosities or associated with distension of the main venous trunk (palpate the GSV in the thigh and the LSV in the calf if they are not visible)? The LSV is deep to the deep fascia and so is usually difficult to see even if grossly distended, but it can be felt.
  - congested veins (not varicose) cause a blue discolouration to the leg, particularly when the skin venules are affected and may be confused with bruising.
- Look for leg swelling, comparing the two legs. Is it compressible or non-compressible (usually indicates lymphoedema)? How far up does it go?
- Look for skin changes in the gaiter area (just above the malleoli) (Fig. 3.2):
  - brown pigmentation due to haemosiderin deposits from breakdown of extravasated red blood cells;
  - eczema—may also occur in small patches over more prominent varicosities elsewhere;
  - lipodermatosclerosis—thickening and contraction of the skin producing the 'inverted beer bottle' leg;
  - atrophie blanche—pale patch of skin containing telangiectases, may also occur below the malleoli and on the foot;
  - ulceration—usually medial (in association with GSV incompetence), but may be lateral (with LSV incompetence) and can spread circumferentially.
- Check foot pulses and, if absent, measure ABPIs. Compression is commonly used in treatment but should be avoided if there is significant arterial disease (ABPI < 0.85). The foot pulses may be absent in 'phlegmasia alba dolens' ('the white leg of pregancy') where extensive acute pelvic vein thrombosis impairs venous outflow to the extent that arterial inflow is impaired.
- If there remains doubt about venous incompetence after inspection, insonate with a Doppler probe over the sapheno-femoral and sapheno-popliteal junctions whist squeezing the thigh or calf, respectively. The Doppler probe will detect venous flow upwards with compression (normal) but will also detect any reflux in the superficial vein on relaxing the squeeze. It is not possible to differentiate between popliteal vein and LSV reflux with this method.

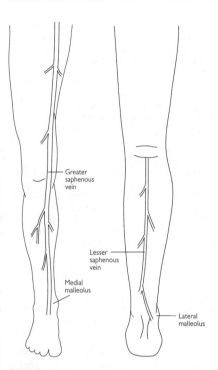

Fig. 3.1 Greater and lesser saphenous systems of veins.

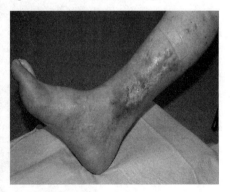

Fig. 3.2 Venous ulcer.

- If considering intervention beyond compression hose then you need to identify the site(s) of incompetence and, in certain patients (those with any history to suggest DVT, those with recurrent varicose veins, or those with sudden onset of varicose disease in middle age onwards), any coexistent deep venous disease.
  - The Doppler probe, used as above, is useful in confirming reflux at the SFJ prior to a first time sapheno-femoral ligation and stripping and, if there is no reflux in the popliteal fossa or suspicion of deep venous disease, may be all that is required. It cannot:
    — differentiate between deep and superficial reflux in the popliteal fossa;
    — provide detailed information on the deep veins;
    — reliably identify incompetent calf perforating veins.
  - Duplex ultrasonography may be available in clinic and can be used to confirm incompetence in either GSV or LSV and to interrogate the deep system up to the IVC if necessary to document the extent of any incompetence (widespread deep venous incompetence probably reduces the effectiveness of intervention for superficial incompetence) and the presence of any obstruction (which is probably a contraindication for superficial venous intervention).
- Lie the patient down and examine the abdomen for:
  - distended abdominal wall veins—these develop to provide a collateral circulation when the iliac veins are obstructed;
  - lower abdominal mass;
  - lower abdominal tenderness suggesting inflammation.
- If a high degree of suspicion then vaginal or rectal examination of the pelvis may be necessary but often pelvic ultrasound or CT scan is more productive.

Differential diagnosis on examination

Leg swelling
- Lymphoedema produces a brawny non-pitting oedema that affects the toes much more than swelling due to venous disease.
- Congestive cardiac failure is usually associated with a raised JVP and at least basal crepitations on chest auscultation.
- Hypoproteinaemia due to liver disease is likely to be associated with other signs of liver disease.

Acute painful calf swelling Ruptured Baker's cyst produces marked tenderness in the upper calf.

Investigation of arterial and venous disease

Overview

Investigation of the circulatory system comprises not only imaging of diseased blood vessels but also measurement of blood flow, velocity, and pressures. The planning of imaging and tests in vascular surgery follows the general principle of using non-invasive methods first followed by invasive methods only if necessary when intervention is being considered.

A great deal of information can be derived from duplex scanning and this is often enough to accurately delineate disease and plan treatment. CT- and MR-angiography are useful adjuncts where technical problems or vessel calcification limit the information from duplex scanning.

The role of transfemoral angiography as a purely diagnostic technique is gradually diminishing as other techniques improve resolution and reliability in detecting disease and providing information for planning treatment.

The non-invasive vascular laboratory

Doppler

- The Doppler probe emits high frequency sound waves that, with the probe placed on the body surface, are reflected off flowing blood (mainly red cells). Movement of the reflective surface causes a frequency shift that depends on the blood flow velocity and the angle of interrogation and is recorded by a transducer in the probe.
- Hand-held (continuous wave) Doppler gives semi-quantitative information on flow, which it emits as an audible signal. Normal arteries produce a good volume biphasic or triphasic signal (Fig. 4.1). The triphasic signal arises when the pressure wave arrives at the insonated artery significantly later than at upstream vessels so that the flow reverses transiently, producing the second phase followed by restored forward flow. If the pressure delay is less marked then it produces a biphasic signal. Monophasic signal is associated with an upstream stenosis that prevents reverse flow and delays the time to peak flow.

Ankle brachial pressure index (ABPI)

- This compares the supine ankle pressure in the AT and PT arteries to the brachial pressure, measured using an upper arm cuff and a Doppler probe over the brachial artery (Fig. 4.2).
- Brachial pressures are usually assumed to be equal in the two arms but occasionally upper limb arterial disease reduces the pressure on one side; in these circumstances use the arm with the higher pressure.
- A standard arm cuff is used on both arm and ankles. Hold the Doppler probe at 45° to the surface where maximum signal is obtained. Inflate the cuff, keeping your eyes on the probe: a slight movement here will cause signal loss. Once the signal disappears, move your attention to the pressure reading and deflate the cuff, recording the pressure at which the signal disappears.
- The ankle pressure is divided by the brachial pressure. Values less than 0.9 indicate a significant stenosis.

Ankle brachial pressure index

> 0.9 Normal
> 0.5 Compatible with claudication alone
< 0.5 Compatible with rest pain and ischaemic tissue necrosis

---

- Arterial calcification makes the arteries incompressible and produces a falsely elevated ankle pressure. This is a particular problem in patients with diabetes and renal failure.
- The pole test can be used to measure ankle pressure in patients with non-compressible (calcified) vessels. Measure the vertical height above the heart at which the Doppler signal over the pedal arteries disappears and convert this to mmHg (77cm water (blood) = 100mmHg).

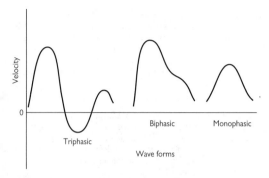

Fig. 4.1 Doppler waveforms recorded over a peripheral artery.

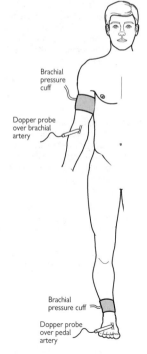

Fig. 4.2 Measuring ankle brachial pressure index.

Exercise test

Patients with long distance claudication (300m+) may have a normal ABPI at rest. Do an exercise test either by asking the patient to step on and off a stool 10 times or to walk for 1min on a treadmill at 4kph and 10% incline and remeasure the ankle pressure with the patient supine as soon as possible after stopping exercise. A drop of > 15mmHg indicates significant arterial stenosis upstream.

Duplex scanning

- Duplex uses a combination of pulsed wave Doppler and ultrasound imaging. Measurement of the reflected waves and their wavelength allows the direction and velocity of blood flow to be determined. The pulsed wave allows the sample volume to be defined so that the signal can be accurately collected from a specific vessel selected on the ultrasound-generated image.
- A significant increase in arterial flow velocity indicates stenosis.
- Dependent duplex (performed with the legs hanging down off the side of the bed) may be useful in visualizing the run-off arteries in the foot when considering distal bypass grafting. It can be more sensitive than angiography in picking up low flow in these distal vessels.
- Duplex using distal manual compression and Valsalva manoeuvres can accurately map reflux and competence in the superficial and deep venous systems as well as demonstrating obstruction.

Other methods of measuring venous function

Also see reference 1.

Plethysmography

Some vascular laboratories use plethysmography to measure changes in leg volume during and after exercise. These changes reflect mainly changes in venous volume and can generate measurements such as 'expelled volume' (with exercise) and refilling time (after exercise). Tourniquets can be applied higher in the leg to demonstrate the contribution of superficial venous reflux to refilling time.

Ambulatory venous pressure

This is an invasive technique in which a needle is placed in a foot on the dorsum of the foot and used to measure pressure changes during and after a standard exercise. The maximum drop in pressure with exercise and the refilling time after exercise can be measured. As with plethysmography, the effect of tourniquet control of superficial venous reflux on these measurements can also be assessed (Fig. 4.3).

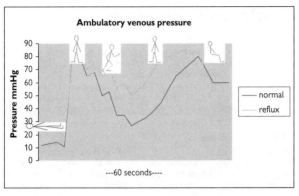

Fig. 4.3 Ambulatory venous pressure.

Radiological investigations

X-ray

- Plain X-rays have a limited role in vascular imaging but can often demonstrate calcified arterial walls and in this way may (usually incidentally) reveal aneurysmal disease.
- X-ray of the infected foot is a useful initial investigation in checking for osteomyelitis (Fig. 4.4). A normal appearance does not rule out bone infection, however, and, if there is a high index of suspicion clinically, follow up with MRI.

CT/CT angiography

Computerized tomography (CT) using spiral multislice scanners is playing an increasing role in vascular imaging. Vascular structures are enhanced using intravenous contrast to produce CT angiography. This technique demands relatively high volume contrast loads and should be avoided if renal function is precarious.

MRI/MR angiography

Magnetic resonance imaging (MRI) gives high quality soft tissue imaging without using radiation. Blood flow can be imaged in MR arteriography (MRA) or MR venography (MRV) by using specific pulse sequences or by injecting gadolinium contrast. MR images are distorted by metal implants, e.g. stents.

Conventional arteriography

- Images are obtained by injecting iodinated contrast medium through a catheter positioned in the arterial system.
- Access is usually gained through the common femoral artery; the brachial approach is less common.
- Retrograde arteriography is performed by passing the catheter up to the abdominal aorta and imaging all downstream arteries after intra-aortic contrast injection.
- Antegrade arteriography involves downward passage of the catheter from the CFA to produce high quality distal images with lower contrast load when the aorto-iliac segment is known to be patent (e.g. on duplex).
- Digital subtraction images are produced by computerized subtraction of a precontrast image from the angiogram images. This removes bony detail and leaves a clear picture of the arterial tree.
- Endovascular procedures of angioplasty, stenting, and coiling can be performed as indicated.
- After catheter withdrawal the arterial puncture site is sealed with compression or a closure device that seals the puncture site with absorbable collagen.

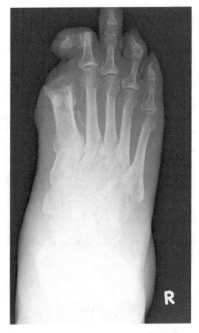

Fig. 4.4 Osteomyelitis in the distal 1st metatarsal following amputation of the first toe.

Blood tests

Whilst work up will be tailored for the individual patient, the following blood tests are of general relevance to the vascular patients and should be performed at some stage.

- Haemoglobin—anaemia and polycythaemia are both relevant findings.
- Platelet count—if < 50,000 patient will need platelet packs for surgery. A high platelet count is associated with increased peripheral thrombosis.
- Renal function (urea, creatinine, potassium) may be impaired because of renal artery atherosclerosis. Use contrast agents with caution in such cases.
- Coagulation screen.
  - APTT, PT/INR as screening tests before conventional arteriography or surgery.
  - D-dimer levels elevated with acute DVT.
  - Factor V Leiden, protein C and S, antithrombin, lupus anticoagulant used to screen for pro-coagulant status, particularly in DVT.
- Lipids—HDL/LDL cholesterol.
- Glucose.
- Thyroid function tests if any clinical suspicion of abnormality.

Cardiac investigations

See also Chapter 7.
- ECG—essential before any surgical intervention and often useful when searching for an embolic source (AF or MI).
- Echocardiography.
  - Ventricular function at rest and with stress (exercise or pharmacological vasodilatation) to assess myocardial risk with major surgery.
  - To search for intracardiac embolic source.
- Coronary angiography performed as a prelude to major vascular surgery when there is evidence of reversible myocardial ischaemia with stress. Stenting can be performed at the same time and the potential for CABG assessed if necessary.

Reference

1 Nicolaides AN (2000). Investigation of chronic venous insufficiency. A consensus statement. *Circulation* **102**, e126–63.

Non-operative treatment of arterial and venous disease

Arterial disease: introduction and investigation

- It is now clear that intermittent claudication is a marker of global atherosclerotic disease and the 10-year mortality from cardiovascular causes is 50%. Thus the most important aspect of the management of patients with peripheral arterial occlusive disease (PAOD) is the assessment and aggressive management of their modifiable risk factors.
- As part of the clinical assessment of patients with PAOD a specific history of the risk factors and associations must be undertaken. These are outlined in the boxes.
- An essential part of the assessment of claudicants is the degree of handicap experienced by them and the extent to which their disability affects their lifestyle and quality of life.
- The examination of patients should include a general examination as well as full cardiovascular examination. In particular, the patient's weight, height, and blood pressure should be recorded.

Risk factors for PAOD
- Tobacco smoking
- Hypertension
- Diabetes mellitus
- Hypercholesterolaemia
- Family history

Factors associated with PAOD but not proven to be risk factors
- Obesity
- Diet
- Sedentary lifestyle
- Gender
- Occupation

Investigation
- The investigation should include laboratory blood tests (p. 66) as well as ECG and ABPI.
- An objective assessment of disability using either a treadmill or corridor-walking test is helpful as a baseline.
- Assessment of the handicap or quality of life using either a linear analogue scale or Short Form 36 (SF-36) has been used mainly to demonstrate the effect of different treatments. In practice asking patients to list those activities restricted by their symptoms may be just as useful.
- A good disease-specific quality of life tool for claudicants is unavailable.

Basic management of arterial disease

It is important to spend time explaining the systemic nature of vascular disease to the patient, in particular the coexistence of coronary artery, cerebrovascular, and peripheral arterial disease. The significant risk reduction of cardiovascular events produced by aggressive risk factor modification needs to be clearly conveyed to the patient. The modifiable risk factors for each patient should be identified and addressed in turn. Table 5.1 outlines the modifiable risk factors and the appropriate strategy for each. In the past the approach has been to advise a combination of stop smoking, keep walking, and take an aspirin. There is now a wealth of evidence supporting a more aggressive approach.

- Advice only to stop smoking results in 1% success, the addition of nicotine replacement therapy increases this to 6%, and early reports using bupropion with counselling appear to increase this to an 18% 1-year success rate.
- For hypertensive patients the aim should be to control blood pressure to a level below 140mmHg systolic and 85mmHg diastolic with appropriate agents. Regular blood pressure monitoring in the community with these targets has been shown to decrease cardiovascular event rate. For the more difficult patient specialist referral is advised.
- The National Service Framework Guidelines for cardiovascular disease prevention advise cholesterol lowering to below 5.0mmol/L with a statin. There is now good evidence that this strategy results in a significant risk reduction. In fact, a 20% reduction in the cholesterol level regardless of the baseline level in patients with evidence of atherosclerotic disease results in a significant risk reduction in cardiovascular events.
- For diabetic patients both good control of diabetes and modification of the above risk factors result in increased patient survival and reduced morbidity.
- The use of antiplatelet therapy in further risk reduction is well documented with aspirin and there is now evidence for the efficacy of clopidogrel in achieving the same risk reduction.
- There is little objective evidence for other lifestyle modification such as exercise, dietary manipulation, and weight reduction in reducing cardiac risk. However, exercise does have a positive impact on symptoms and thus remains a recommendation. Exercise programmes have proven as effective as angioplasty in relieving the symptoms of PAOD but not with a survival benefit. There is now mounting evidence that truncal obesity may be an independent risk factor for atherosclerosis.
- The use of vascular nurse specialists for lifestyle modification advice and supervised exercise programmes has been popular with patients. This may in part be due to the extra time nurses can provide for patient education. A number of centres have joint risk factor management clinics with interested physicians and vascular surgeons working side by side.

Table 5.1 Strategy for modifiable risk factors

Risk factor	Strategy
Smoking	Smoking cessation: advice; nicotine replacement; counselling; bupropion
Hypertension	Antihypertensive therapy, aiming for BP < 140/85mmHg
Hypercholesterolaemia	Statin therapy aiming for cholesterol < 5.0mmol/L
Diabetes mellitus	Dietary manipulation & oral hypoglycaemics or insulin aiming for postprandial peak glucose 7.6–9mmol/L
Vascular disease	Antiplatelet therapy: aspirin 75mg or clopidogrel 75mg if aspirin contraindicated
Obesity	Dietary manipulation, weight reduction, increased exercise
Sedentary lifestyle	Exercise programme (with or without supervision)

Exercise programmes

Supervised exercise programmes have the most sustained effect. Most meet for 1–2 hours on a weekly basis and involve warm-up exercises followed by brisk walking. The main benefit seems to be from peer support of meeting regularly and exercising as a group. For many patients just simply walking for 20–30min each day has the same effect and this is all that is needed for highly motivated patients, particularly if travel to a supervised programme is an issue. Supervised exercise programmes have been shown to double the claudication and maximum walking distances in up to 3/4 of patients within 6 months.

Other interventions

The decision on which other interventions to offer the patient will depend on the balance between benefit to the patient of the intervention proposed and the risks inherent with the intervention. The degree to which claudication restricts specific activities and the importance of those activities are crucial in the discussion with the patient over treatment choice.

- The other non-surgical interventions available to patients include angioplasty, angioplasty with stenting, sympathectomy (chemical or operative), and prostacyclin infusions. Most other medical treatments for symptomatic relief do not have a robust evidence base to support their widespread use. The most important of these options for patients with claudication is angioplasty and/or stenting.
- Drug therapy for symptomatic relief in claudicants has been disappointing and over the last decade has been superseded by risk factor modification and exercise programmes or percutaneous interventions. Cilostazol does have a licence for symptomatic treatment of claudication and is part of the protocol for a number of centres. It needs to be used in conjunction with risk factor modification and the cost of it compared to exercise is difficult to justify. It may be of some use in providing initial symptomatic benefit whilst motivating patients to exercise.
- Sympathectomy and prostacyclin infusion are reserved mainly for those with un-reconstructable critical limb ischaemia who decline amputation. Most centres have moved away from open or laparoscopic lumbar sympathectomy, although chemical sympathectomy (transcutaneous approach to the lumbar sympathetic chain under X-ray screening followed by phenol injection of the chain) may be of use when there is significant rest pain but little tissue loss. Like prostacyclin infusions, it may also be useful for the management of patients with vasculitis, microangiopathy (e.g. in diabetics), or severe vasospastic disease without large vessel disease.

Angioplasty and/or stenting

This has revolutionized the treatment of claudicants over the past 15 years. It has virtually abolished the need for operative bypass in the aorto-iliac segments with good medium-term results. It has superseded surgery for claudicants with disease in the femoral artery with the exception of localized disease of the common femoral artery where surgery is still the preferred treatment option.

The advent of subintimal angioplasty of the superficial femoral artery has also resulted in a dramatic reduction in the numbers of infrainguinal bypass procedures. Even in the tibial vessels (below knee calf vessels) many centres are reporting good results that threaten to make infrainguinal bypass surgery obsolete for even short distance claudication and critical ischaemia.

The long-term results of angioplasty and stenting, however, are not clear and a number of trials have shown that, even as early as 18 months, the outcome for supervised exercise programmes is equivalent to that for angioplasty for SFA disease.

The risks of angioplasty and stenting include an overall 5% risk of bleeding, haematoma, or false aneurysm with a 1% risk of urgent surgery and a 0.1% risk of limb loss. Despite this they are an important treatment option as they provide early symptomatic improvement for patients and obviate the higher risks of surgery for patients with claudication alone as an indication.

Deciding on intervention

Best practice is for the treatment options, each with a risk–benefit assessment, to be made and discussed with the patient, allowing them to make an informed choice. This allows a tailormade treatment plan for each patient taking into account their co-morbidity and lifestyle limitations arising from the extent of their disease.

Regular joint meetings with the interventional radiologists to discuss all patients undergoing interventions and a process of peer review of cases allow high standards to be maintained. Ongoing unit data collection on numbers undergoing interventions and their outcome will allow an accurate assessment of risks/benefits to patients in individual institutions.

Venous disease: introduction

A number of alternative interventions to conventional open surgery for varicose veins have recently become available. These offer the potential for treatment without general anaesthesia or in-patient stay and with more rapid recovery. These newer techniques may replace ligation or stripping of the greater or lesser saphenous systems, or removal of superficial varicosities, or both.

Radiofrequency catheter ablation (OPCS code L94)

This technique relies on occlusion of the greater saphenous vein using radiofrequency energy to induce resistive heating of the vein wall. The procedure may be performed under local or general anaesthetic. It provides an alternative to sapheno-femoral ligation and stripping.

Procedure
- The GSV is cannulated under duplex ultrasound guidance just above or below the knee.
- Using the Seldinger technique, a guidewire is passed proximally.
- The radiofrequency catheter is introduced over the wire into the GSV and passed proximally so the tip lies just beyond the sapheno-femoral junction.
- Saline mixed with local anaesthetic is now infiltrated along the length of the vein under ultrasound guidance in the intrafascial plane. This serves both as anaesthetic and to insulate the vein from surrounding tissues, and also compresses the vein.
- The electrodes at the tip of the catheter are deployed so that they are in contact with the vein wall and the catheter is energized.
- Radiofrequency energy passes into the vein wall and is converted into heat, which causes the vessel wall to shrink.
- The catheter is slowly drawn along the length of the vein at 1mm every 2–3sec.
- Ultrasonography confirms occlusion of the vessel at the end of the procedure. If this has not been achieved, the procedure may be repeated immediately providing the catheter can be re-passed.
- Stab avulsions of superficial varicosities may be carried out at the time of the procedure.

Follow-up
Compression hosiery (class II) is worn from immediately after the procedure for at least 1 week. Any residual flow in the GSV at 6 weeks can be treated by injection of sclerosant. Residual superficial varicosities can be treated by sclerosant injection or multiple avulsion phlebectomies under local or general anaesthetic. RFA has been used to treat the LSV but few data are available.

Complications

- Bruising, haematoma, oedema are relatively common.
- Burn injuries to the common femoral vein can occur if the catheter is inadvertently advanced into the deep vein, with concomitant risk of DVT (2%).
- Burns to the subcutaneous tissues can be sustained if there is inadequate local anaesthetic fluid insulating the vein (0.5%). If this involves the saphenous nerve, paraesthesia may result (2%).

Outcome

- Immediate successful closure of GSV in 88–100% of patients.
- GSV remains closed in 85–90% at 4 years.
- Rates of recurrence and neovascularization: clinical improvement similar to that with conventional surgery at 2 years.
- No long-term data.

Endovenous laser therapy (EVLT; OPCS code L94)

Procedure

Technique similar to radiofrequency catheter ablation, but with closure of the vein achieved using a diode laser, 810 or 940nm wavelength. This is introduced into the vein in the same way, under ultrasound guidance. Lidocaine 0.1% is infiltrated around the vein. EVLT can be carried out more rapidly, with the laser catheter withdrawn at a rate of 10mm every 3sec while the laser is firing. The procedure can be carried out under local or general anaesthetic.

Follow-up Class II compression hosiery is worn continuously from the time of the procedure for at least a week. Residual varicosities at 6 weeks can be treated as per radiofrequency ablation.

Complications

- Superficial phlebitis is common in tributaries.
- Bruising over the treated vein, though uncommon.
- Saphenous nerve paraesthesia—uncommon.
- Skin burns have only been reported with higher powered (1064nm) lasers.
- DVT.

Outcome

- Initial success in GSV closure of 94–100%.
- GSV remains closed in 98% of limbs at 5 years.
- No long-term follow-up data is available.

Foam sclerotherapy

Procedure

- The vein to be treated (GSV or LSV) is cannulated under duplex-guidance after infiltration of the skin with local anaesthetic.
- Foam sclerosant is generated by the combination of either sodium tetradecyl sulphate (STD) 1–3% or the detergent polidocanol 0.5–3% with air in the ratio 1:3–4. This can be achieved mixing air with sclerosant vigorously in two syringes connected by a three-way tap.
- With the leg elevated, 6–8mL of foam is injected into the vein under duplex imaging. Displacement of blood from the vein causes immediate spasm.
  - Progression of foam proximally is observed by ultrasound. Ultrasound-guided compression of the SFJ or SPJ is applied as the foam approaches the junction to prevent foam entering the deep system.
  - Foam may be milked distally into superficial varicosities to treat these also.
  - Additional superficial varicosities may be cannulated separately and injected with foam or liquid sclerosant.
- The limb is immediately placed in compression bandaging and class II compression hosiery, which should remain undisturbed for 1–2 weeks.
- Some patients will require one or two further treatments.

Complications

- Thrombophlebitis (5%).
- DVT as a result of extension of thrombus from the treated vein into the deep system (< 1%).
- Visual disturbance (2%)—flashing light or blurring of vision. Usually transient, resolving within a few hours. More common in patients with history of migraine.
- Transient cough.
- TIA and CVA—theoretical risk in presence of patent septal defect.
- Skin pigmentation—common initially (25%, but fades in most cases).
- Skin necrosis may result from extravasation of sclerosant. Less likely with polidocanol than STD.
- Allergic reaction to sclerosant—rare.

Outcome

- 80% of GSVs remain occluded at 3 years. 97% of superficial varicosities have been abolished.
- No long-term data available.

Other interventions for venous disease

Liquid sclerotherapy

Used to treat superficial varicosities.

Procedure

- With the patient standing, superficial varicosities are cannulated with 25G short butterfly needles at a number of sites, ensuring that blood can be withdrawn to confirm placement of the needle in the vessel lumen. The butterflies are taped in place.
- The patient lies down and the leg is elevated to empty the vein.
- A small quantity of sclerosant (usually STD 1–3%) is injected at each site, the cannula removed, and local compression applied using a dental roll or piece of foam secured with tape.
- Once all sites have been treated, the leg is bandaged while still elevated, usually with a cohesive bandage firmly applied, covered with class II compression hosiery. This is removed after 3 weeks.
- The procedure may be repeated as necessary.

Complications

- Skin necrosis if sclerosant extravasates or if cannula is not within the vein lumen (< 5%).
- Skin pigmentation (25%)—may be permanent.
- Bruising.
- Thrombophlebitis.
- Matting—formation of network of tiny veins over injection site.

Microsclerotherapy Similar technique to that of liquid sclerotherapy. Fine needles are used to inject sclerosant into thread veins or telangiectases.

Laser therapy Laser energy is directly applied to thread veins and telangiectases through the skin. May cause hyper- or hypopigmentation at the site.

Microwave thermocoagulation Used in the treatment of thread veins and telangiectasia. Microwave energy is applied via a fine needle introduced directly into the vessel to coagulate the blood.

Management of complex leg ulcers

Leg ulcers in the diabetic patient

The prevalence of type II diabetes is increasing. Atherosclerosis is a common complication of diabetes. Diabetics are at risk of ulceration due to neuropathic and ischaemic complications of diabetes. The presence of neuropathy and microvascular disease requires a more complex management strategy than that for the patient with pure occlusive vascular disease.

Assessment

The diabetic foot can be assessed simply and straightforwardly by focused history and examination employing inspection, palpation, and sensory testing. Although some specialized equipment, such as a neurothesiometer, toe pressure machine, or transcutaneous oxygen tension machine, can be useful, they are not essential.

Ischaemia

- Lower limb and foot pulses.
- Colour, temperature, capillary refill time.
- Tissue loss or ulceration.
- Doppler pressures.

The ABPI measured by a cuff is unreliable in patients with medial arterial calcification. Pressure measurement by measuring height above heart at which Doppler signal over pedal arteries is extinguished is accurate (77cm water (blood) = 100mmHg).

Neuropathy

Neuropathy may delay the presentation of ischaemia because the patient does not have pain.

Motor

- High medial arch.
- Prominent metatarsal heads.

Autonomic

- Dry skin with fissuring.
- Decreased sweating.
- Distended veins (AV shunting).

Sensory

- Light touch with cotton wisp.
- 10g nylon monofilament.
- Vibration—128Hz tuning fork.

Deformity

- Clawed toes.
- Pes cavus.
- Hallux rigidus.
- Hallux valgus.
- Hammer toe.
- Charcot foot:
  - rocker bottom deformity;
  - medial convexity.

- Nail deformity.
- Previous amputations or surgery.

Callus
- At sites of high pressure and friction.

Swelling/oedema
- Concomitant cardiac failure.
- Renal impairment.
- Venous insufficiency.
- Lymphoedema.
- Gout.
- AV shunting.
- Infection.
- Charcot foot.

Skin breakdown
- Especially between the toes.
- Back of the heel.
- Bullae/blisters.

Infection
- Erythema.
- Swelling.
- Warmth.
- Fluctuation.
- Discharge.
- Discolouration.

Necrosis
- Black or brown devitalized tissue.

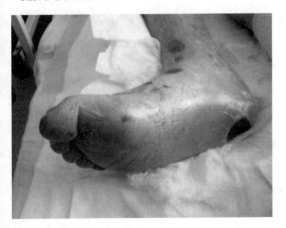

Fig. 6.1 Distorted foot in peripheral neuropathy.

Management of leg ulcers in the diabetic patient

Good management requires a multidisciplinary team. A diabetic foot clinic brings together the expertise of the various members of the team and has been shown to improve outcomes and reduce amputation rates. The core team comprises diabetic physician, podiatrist, nurse, and orthotist with visits from vascular surgeons and orthopaedic surgeons. The vascular surgeon's contibution is to decide when revascularization is required and how to achieve it. Surgery may be to drain infection, debride, amputate, stabilize, or revascularize and it is often incumbent on the vascular surgeon to operate on these patients.

The neuropathic foot

The blood supply is adequate; foot pulses are present. Debridement is usually carried out by the podiatrist in a clinic setting. An ulcer should be debrided by removing all surrounding callus, cutting away all slough and non-viable tissue, a deep swab taken for culture, the wound cleaned with sterile saline, and a sterile dressing applied with a bandage. Pressure-relieving footwear is required. The wound should be reviewed at weekly intervals and the debridement repeated.

Osteomyelitis

If the ulcer probes to bone or bone is exposed then infection of the bone is likely. If osteomyelitis is proven on plain X-rays or MRI scan or the ulcer fails to heal by 3 months despite regular debridement, excision of the underlying bone is usually required to heal the ulcer. Occasionally a prolonged course of appropriate antibiotics (e.g. clindamycin) will heal osteomyelitis in a phalange (or a terminal phalange may be extruded), avoiding the need for surgery.

Neuroischaemic ulcer

- If the Doppler pressure is 100mmHg or more revascularization is not required and debridement can proceed as described above for the neuropathic foot.
- If the Doppler pressure is 50mmHg or less revascularization will be required to heal the ulcer or any partial foot amputation. Revascularization should aim for 'in line' vascular continuity into the foot. If this is not possible or it fails, a major amputation will be required. Postponing amputation in this situation only delays the inevitable with ongoing disabilty for the patient.
- A foot with an ankle Doppler pressure between 50 and 100mmHg may require revascularization and the individual case needs to be treated according to its merits. A period of time may make it clear if the ulceration is healing. If a straightforward (low risk) angioplasty is possible, then early intervention is probably justified but if the disease is in the crural arteries, the risk of angioplasty increases especially if there is only single vessel run-off from the angioplasty site. Increasing numbers of interventional radiologists have expertise in crural subintimal angioplasty, which can be successful. The alternative is a distal bypass graft.

Distal bypass surgery

Diabetic patients often have patent popliteal arteries but occlusive disease of the crural vessels. Visualization of the arteries into the foot, i.e. the dorsalis pedis and posterior tibial arteries and their branches, is necessary at angiography if a bypass on to a distal tibial or tarsal vessel is being considered. Information on the run-off into the foot may also be predicted by dependent Doppler and duplex scanning or magnetic resonanance angiography. Absence of a plantar arch or vascular calcification is not considered to be a contraindication to reconstruction, nor is a stenosis downstream to the anastomosis of less than 50%. Autologous vein is required. The popliteal artery can sometimes be used for the proximal anastomosis to keep the graft short and reduce the length of vein required. If there is an isolated popliteal segment the composite sequential technique can be employed using a prosthetic from the femoral to the above knee popliteal and autologous vein taken from here to the distal anastomosis.

Necrosis and infection

Collections of pus or wet necrosis should be drained and debrided as a matter of urgency. Do not wait until after angiography. The full extent of tissue loss may not be apparent until formal operative debridement is underway. Larval therapy may be useful as an adjunct here when debridement alone is needed. Once all devitalized tissue has been removed, consideration should be given to how a useful healed foot can be achieved. Once important weight-bearing parts of the hindfoot are missing, the foot is beyond salvage. The use of the vacuum-assisted closure dressing system and subsequent plastic surgical reconstruction has extended the possibilities in foot salvage.

Antibiotics

Clinical signs of infection can be diminished in the diabetic patient and untreated infection often leads rapidly to necrosis and major amputation. Broad spectrum empirical antibiotics are therefore employed until swab results are obtained. (e.g. amoxicillin, flucloxacillin, and metronidazole) It is important that a deep tissue swab/tissue is sent after initial debridement as the surface organisms are unlikely to be representative. Isolated Gram-negative organisms should not be assumed to be commensals and need to be treated with appropriate antibiotics. See Chapter 10.

Ulceration associated with mixed arterial and venous disease of the leg

Patients with venous disease of the leg often have recurrent gaiter area ulceration over many years, which usually responds to compression treatment. They may, however, reach a stage where a recurrent ulcer is more painful than previously, especially on elevation, and compression treatment is difficult to tolerate and leads to a deterioration in the ulcer. This marks the advent of significant arterial disease that is compromising ulcer healing. Compression can cause limb loss and must be avoided. It is essential, therefore, that pulses and, if necessary, ABPIs are reassessed with each new 'venous' ulcer. The degree of arterial compromise dictates the management strategy.

Patient assessment

Arterial disease
- Pain on elevation or with compression bandaging.
- Atypical ulceration for pure venous disease.
- Tissue loss on the foot.
- Loss of pulses.
- ABPI.
- Beware coexisting diabetes mellitus.
- ABPI by elevation if stiff or calcified arteries.
- Duplex scanning.
- Arteriography.

Venous disease
- Previous venous ulceration.
- Old DVT.
- New DVT in patient with known arterial disease.
- Varicose veins.
- Poor gaiter skin, especially lipodermatosclerosis.
- Duplex scanning to assess extent and cause of chronic venous disease and suitable vein for bypass graft.
- Occasionally MRV or conventional venography are needed to assess extent of venous disease.

Management
- If the ABPI is > 0.85 then it is safe to proceed with standard high compression bandaging (or venous surgery).
- A group with moderate arterial insufficiency can be defined by an ABPI of 0.5–0.85. These patients can have a trial of modified compression aiming for a pressure of 30mmHg at the ankle by reducing the stretch on the bandages to 25% extension or missing out one layer. These patients need to be reviewed and the strategy changed to the same as that of the severe group if there are adverse effects:
  - increasing ulcer size;
  - development of rest pain;
  - failure to improve after 3 months.

- The severe group with an ABPI of < 0.5 should be considered for revascularization.
  - If followed by elevation and compression this will often lead to ulcer healing.
  - Even if there is superficial venous incompetence, the GSV or LSV is often a good size and suitable as a conduit if necessary with plication of one or two varicose 'blow outs'. **It is therefore prudent not to rush to venous surgery in these patients without considering the need for concurrent or future arterial bypass surgery.**
  - The strategy for arterial reconstruction is otherwise the same as for patients with pure arterial disease. After successful revascularization (angioplasty or bypass graft), compression may be applied providing the arterial graft is not in a superficial location.
  - If revascularization is not possible, fails, or is insufficient, the ulcer may be healed with a period of bed rest and elevation but this will require adequate pain control with analgesics (regular morphine if necessary) or an epidural.
  - Even with successful revascularization the ulcers may take a long time to heal; 6 months is typical. Skin grafting is a way of rapidly achieving skin cover with either split skin or pinch grafts.

Perioperative management of ischaemic heart disease

Coronary risk of peripheral vascular surgery

Coronary artery disease is important to the vascular surgeon for two reasons.

- Obstructive coronary disease is very common in patients with peripheral vascular disease.
- Peripheral vascular operations are often major procedures associated with significant cardiovascular stress.

Of patients with abdominal aortic aneurysms, carotid disease, or lower limb ischaemia:

- history suggests coronary disease in > 50%;
- significant angiographic coronary disease in > 60%.

Postoperative myocardial infarction

- Common following peripheral vascular surgery:
  - diagnostic rise in serum troponin in 5–10%;
  - minor rise in troponin in an additional 10–30%.
- Mortality rate 30–50%, 3–4 times that of spontaneous MI.
- Main cause of cardiac death, which accounts for 50% of perioperative mortality.
- Only slightly less common in infrainguinal versus abdominal aortic surgery, although carotid surgery carries a much lower risk.

Coronary risk following peripheral vascular surgery

Patients who survive peripheral vascular surgery are at increased risk of coronary events longer term compared to the general population of a similar age.

- 1 year mortality 10–20%.

Pathophysiology of perioperative myocardial infarction

Spontaneous out-of-hospital acute MI:
- rupture of vulnerable atheromatous plaque;
- subsequent thrombosis and partial or complete coronary occlusion.

Perioperative MI is less well understood, but at autopsy:
- plaque rupture in <50%;
- intracoronary thrombus in 30%.

Supply–demand imbalance is the main factor in most cases of perioperative MI.
- Stress of surgery provokes tachycardia, which peaks on days 1–2.
- Myocardial oxygen demand increases, which in the face of flow-limiting coronary stenoses leads to prolonged myocardial ischaemia with progressive subendocardial necrosis.
- Plaque rupture and thrombosis may occur as a secondary event.
- MI is diagnosed, typically on days 2–3.
- Less commonly, MI occurs within 1–2 days of surgery without warning.

Preoperative assessment: general considerations

'Assessment of cardiac risk' is not an end in itself, but is part of an overall cardiological and surgical management plan aimed at delivering the best possible *overall* prognosis to a given patient, whilst relieving relevant symptoms. Close cooperation between surgeons, anaesthetists, and cardiologists is required, ideally in a multidisciplinary clinic targeted at patients referred for the highest risk operations.

When considering patients for peripheral vascular surgery, a number of issues related to coronary risk should be considered, well in advance of admission.

What is the urgency of surgery?
- If urgent, misplaced concerns about coronary risk can lead to dangerous delays.

What is the coronary risk of the proposed operation?
- For example, carotid endarterectomy is inherently safer than abdominal aortic aneurysm repair.

Does the patient have symptoms of coronary disease (angina)?
- If so, cardiological assessment is indicated independently of the proposed peripheral vascular surgery.

What is the patient-specific risk of a perioperative coronary event?
- If high:
  - should surgery simply be cancelled, or its type modified?
  - is risk-reducing cardiological treatment indicated?

What is the long-term risk of a coronary event following surgery?
- If high:
  - is risk-reducing cardiological treatment indicated?
  - is purely prophylactic vascular surgery appropriate, e.g. repair of an asymptomatic abdominal aortic aneurysm?

Preoperative assessment: clinical factors

50% of patients can be assigned to low or high risk groups based on clinical assessment alone. Similar factors predict both perioperative and long-term cardiac events and presentation to the vascular surgical clinic provides an important opportunity to assess and improve both aspects of risk.

History

Age and sex
- Risk increases with age, particularly over 70 years.
- Risk is similar between the sexes, i.e. protective effect of being female is lost in the vascular surgical population.

Previous cardiac history
- Previous acute coronary syndrome/myocardial infarction.
- Investigation for possible coronary disease within 2 years: if adequate, reassuring, and symptoms stable, reassessment usually unnecessary.
- Percutaneous coronary intervention within 2 years or bypass surgery within 5 years: if symptoms stable, reassessment usually unnecessary.

Symptoms
- Exercise capacity (see Table 7.1): valuable predictor of risk, although many vascular patients limited by non-cardiac factors.
- Angina, suggesting significant obstructive coronary disease.
  - Dull, heavy, tight or squeezing chest pain; may radiate to arms or throat.
  - Provoked by exercise and relieved within a few minutes by rest.
  - More easily provoked after heavy meal.
  - High index of suspicion in high risk vascular surgical population:
    — insufficient exercise to provoke angina regularly;
    — angina may be atypical;
    — exertional dyspnoea may be 'angina-equivalent'.
- Heart failure, suggesting impaired left ventricular function secondary to previous myocardial infarction:
  - exertional dyspnoea;
  - orthopnoea and/or paroxysmal nocturnal dyspnoea;
  - peripheral oedema in biventricular failure.

Coronary risk factors
Aggressive modification is the mainstay of long-term cardiovascular risk reduction.
- Smoking: number of pack-years.
- Hypertension: treatment and control.
- Hypercholesterolaemia: treatment and control.
- Diabetes mellitus: type (1 or 2), treatment (diet alone, oral medication, insulin), control (HbA1c).
- Family history: Important but not modifiable.

Medication
- May have protective effect perioperatively (e.g. beta-blocker).

Table 7.1 Clinical assessment of functional status in metabolic equivalents (METs)*

Number of METS	Can you do the following?
1	Take care of yourself
	Eat, dress, or use the toilet
	Walk indoors around the house
	Walk a block or two on level ground at 2–3mph or 3.2–4.8kph
4	Do light work around the house like dusting or washing dishes
	Climb a flight of stairs or walk up a hill
	Run a short distance
	Do heavy work around the house like scrubbing floors or lifting or moving heavy furniture
	Participate in moderate recreational activities like golf, bowling, dancing, doubles tennis, or throwing a baseball or football
> 10	Participate in strenuous sports like swimming, singles tennis, football, basketball, or skiing

* Adapted from Duke Activity Status Index[1] and AHA Exercise Standards.[2]

Examination

Usually unrewarding in uncomplicated coronary disease, but check the following.
- Blood pressure.
- Signs of heart failure:
  - elevated JVP;
  - displaced apex;
  - third heart sound;
  - crackles at lung bases;
  - peripheral oedema.

Basic investigations

- Fasting lipids and glucose.
  - Identify untreated hypercholesterolaemia or diabetes.
  - Assess adequacy of control on treatment.
- Electrocardiogram.
  - Identify previous infarction (e.g. Q-waves, T-inversion).
  - Baseline for comparison with postoperative recordings.
- PA chest radiograph.
  - Heart size.
  - Evidence of pulmonary congestion.
- Resting echocardiography for left ventricular function.
  - Not routine: does not predict postoperative coronary events.
  - Consider if clinical suggestion of coronary disease or heart failure, because severe left ventricular dysfunction predicts difficult perioperative course and poor long-term survival.

Clinical risk scoring

The absence of any worrying features on routine clinical assessment indicates low perioperative cardiac risk. However, most patients with peripheral vascular disease will have at least one adverse factor, and it is challenging to convert a clinical assessment into a quantifiable risk. Risk scoring systems have been developed based on multivariate analysis of large populations. Many are complex, unwieldy, and difficult to use routinely in a busy clinic. Two simpler systems have been developed (see boxes).

Revised cardiac risk index
- 6 point score.
- For all types of non-cardiac surgery.
- Limited ability to define low-risk group in peripheral vascular surgery as these patients all have minimum score of 1.

Eagle score
- 5 point score.
- Specifically for vascular patients.
- 35% score 0 and can undergo surgery at low risk.
- 15% score > 3 and are at definite high risk; these require formal cardiological assessment prior to surgery.

- 50% score 1–2 and are at an unhelpful 'intermediate' risk; these benefit most from specialized testing with myocardial perfusion scintigraphy or stress echocardiography.

Revised cardiac risk index[3]

Risk factors	Definition
High-risk surgery	AAA repair, thoracic, abdominal
Ischaemic heart disease	MI, Q-waves, nitrates, +ve exercise test
Congestive heart failure	History, examination, chest radiograph
Cerebrovascular disease	Stroke, TIA
Insulin-treated diabetes	
Renal dysfunction	Creatinine > 177µmol/L

Number of factors	Proportion of patients	Cardiac events
0	36%	0.4%
1	39%	1.1%
2	18%	4.6%
3	7%	9.7%

Eagle score[4,5]

Risk factors

- Age ≥ 70
- Diabetes
- Angina
- Myocardial infarction (history or Q-waves)
- Congestive heart failure

Factors	Proportion of patients	LMS/3v CAD*	Events
0	30–40%	5%	3%
1–2	50%	16%	8%
3	10–20%	43%	18%

* Presence of left mainstem or 3-vessel coronary disease at angiography.

Preoperative specialized testing: general considerations

Specialized cardiac testing is expensive and can inadvertently delay important noncardiac surgery. It should be reserved for patients in whom clinical assessment alone gives insufficient reassurance, i.e. those at intermediate risk.

The investigations in common use are:
- exercise electrocardiography (ECG);
- stress–rest myocardial perfusion scintigraphy (MPS);
- stress echocardiography (echo).

These are functional tests that assess the adequacy of myocardial blood supply during stress, in contrast to the anatomical information provided by coronary angiography.

All methods involve two components:
- cardiac stress with exercise or drugs, to provoke relative hypoperfusion of myocardium supplied by stenosed coronary arteries that is not present at rest;
- ECG or imaging, to detect either reduced perfusion or effect of consequent ischaemia on myocardial function.

Exercise ECG is of limited value in:
- patients unable to exercise to an adequate workload (common in vascular surgical population);
- women;
- patients with an abnormal resting ECG.

Exercise testing is often said to be contraindicated in those with abdominal aortic aneurysms, though there is no evidence that it is harmful.

Given the limitations of the exercise ECG, vascular surgical patients are commonly investigated using MPS or stress echo. MPS is a more sensitive method of detecting ischaemia, but the higher specificity of stress echo may be advantageous when only severe coronary disease is of interest. In clinical practice the debate is usually academic, the 'best' technique being the one that is available locally from an expert clinician.

Myocardial perfusion scintigraphy

MPS involves the comparison of images representing relative myocardial perfusion during stress with images representing perfusion at rest.

Cardiac stress

Dynamic exercise stress (treadmill or bicycle) may be used when possible. If not, pharmacological methods are necessary.

- Vasodilators (dipyridamole or adenosine).
  - First choice.
  - Adenosine: direct coronary vasodilatation via A_{2a}-receptors.
  - Dipyridamole: inhibition of breakdown and reuptake of endogenous adenosine, increasing extracellular concentration.
  - Main contraindications: reactive airways disease, unpaced second- or third-degree heart block.
- Inotropes (dobutamine).
  - Synthetic beta-agonist, increasing myocardial oxygen demand with secondary coronary vasodilatation.

Radiopharmaceutical perfusion tracers

A radiopharmaceutical is injected during stress and is taken up by the myocardium in relation to its blood supply.

- Thallium-201 (^{201}Tl).
  - Excellent perfusion tracer physiologically; many years of experience.
  - Immediate post-stress imaging.
  - Redistribution imaging 3–4 hours later for resting perfusion.
  - May be reinjected at rest for optimal detection of viability.
  - Low energy photons and long half-life (73h): soft tissue attenuation problematic; gating difficult; radiation exposure high (± 18mSv).
- Technetium-99m (^{99m}Tc) labelled tracers.
  - ^{99m}Tc-sestamibi or ^{99m}Tc-tetrofosmin.
  - Bind to mitochondria so post-stress imaging can be delayed (e.g. 30–60min post-injection).
  - Separate injection required at rest using 2-day or 1-day protocol.
  - Nitrate may be given prior to resting injection for optimal detection of viability.
  - High energy photons and short half-life (6h): high quality images; gating straightforward (see below); radiation exposure low (± 10mSv).

Imaging

Imaging in MPS is performed using an Anger gamma camera, usually with single-photon emission computed tomography (SPECT).

- Detectors (typically two at 90°) rotate around patient in series of steps (typically 16–32 per head over 180° arc)
- Planar projection acquired at each step, representing distribution of radionuclide within patient.
- Acquisition reconstructed and reorientated to display slices in standard orthogonal planes of the heart.

- Perfusion defects appear as areas of relatively reduced radioactive counts, indicating reduced tracer uptake (Fig. 7.1).
- Regional and global left ventricular function assessed by gating image acquisition to electrocardiogram.

(a)

(b)

(c)

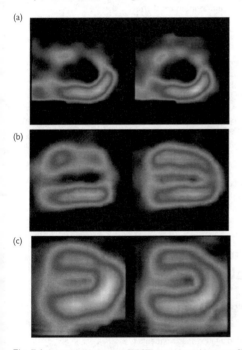

Fig. 7.1 Examples of abnormal SPECT scans. Vertical long-axis SPECT slices from three patients, illustrating three different appearances of the anterior wall. Stress (left) and rest (right) images are shown side by side for comparison. (a) Fixed anterior perfusion defect (seen on both stress and rest acquisitions), suggesting previous infarction. (b) Reversible anterior perfusion defect (seen on stress acquisition only), suggesting flow-limiting coronary stenosis. (c) Anterior attenuation artefact caused by breast tissue in a female patient. Artefacts are common and may be misreported as perfusion defects by the inexperienced.

Stress echocardiography

Stress echo compares myocardial wall motion and thickening at rest and during stress. Considerable skill and experience are required both to obtain good images and to interpret them.

Procedure
- Resting echo is performed, paying careful attention to orientation and quality.
- Important technical refinements.
  - Harmonic imaging provides good image quality in most patients.
  - IV microbubble contrast agents can be used to opacify left ventricular blood pool, allowing clear definition of endocardial border in almost all patients.
  - Digital acquisition of representative cardiac cycle in each standard view allows side-by-side comparison at each level of stress.
- Patient is stressed (see 'Myocardial perfusion scintigraphy', p. 108), most commonly with dobutamine.
- Digital acquisitions repeated at each infusion rate.

Abnormal patterns
- Resting wall motion abnormality suggests infarction.
- New or worsening wall motion abnormality during stress suggests ischaemia, with underlying flow-limiting coronary stenosis.

Clinical value of preoperative functional testing

- Absence of inducible hypoperfusion/ischaemia predicts low risk of postoperative cardiac death or nonfatal MI (1–2%).
- Presence of inducible hypoperfusion/ischaemia more difficult to interpret.
  - Common finding in vascular patients (25–50%).
  - Risk of postoperative cardiac event still 'only' 10–25%.
  - Risk increases with extent of abnormality, but < 50% for even the most ischaemic studies.

It is impossible to identify individuals who will definitely suffer a cardiac event, and a population-based approach is required.
- Focus resources on manageable number of patients with most to gain.
- Define thresholds to trigger further investigation and treatment options, e.g.
  - beta-blockade if *any* ischaemia;
  - coronary angiography (unless clinically indicated) only if extensive ischaemia (> 25% of left ventricular myocardium).

Both MPS and stress echo predict long-term cardiac events following successful surgery. This may be particularly important for patients undergoing peripheral vascular surgery on predominantly prophylactic grounds.

Preoperative strategies for reducing risk

Cardiac stress in the face of flow-limiting coronary stenoses is the main cause of postoperative MI. Preoperative approaches to lowering risk have therefore taken two directions:
- revascularization of stenosed coronary arteries, either by percutaneous coronary intervention (PCI) or coronary artery bypass grafting (CABG);
- pharmacological protection of left ventricular myocardium and vulnerable coronary plaques from stress, e.g. beta-blockade.

Coronary angiography with a view to revascularization

Protective value of revascularization prior to noncardiac surgery

CABG already performed for standard clinical reasons protects against subsequent vascular surgery performed within 5 years. In the Coronary Artery Surgery Study (CASS) registry, risk of death or MI after vascular surgery was found to be:[6]
- no coronary disease, 3%;
- coronary disease managed medically, 11%;
- coronary disease post-CABG, 2%.

PCI *may* be similarly protective, but there are fewer data. In the Bypass Angioplasty Revascularization Investigation (BARI) registry, risk of death or MI after noncardiac surgery was found to be:[7]
- post-CABG, 1.6%;
- post PCI, 1.6%.

It does not follow that revascularization performed solely on the grounds of perioperative risk provides net benefit. In a study on 510 vascular patients (41% AAA) with coronary stenoses on screening (left mainstem excluded), who were randomized to revascularization (PCI 59%, CABG 41%) or medical management, no differences in perioperative or long-term cardiac outcome were found.[8]

Coronary revascularization can only be recommended prior to peripheral vascular surgery if it would have been performed anyway on clinical grounds (e.g. for angina, or for three-vessel/left mainstem disease with demonstrable ischaemia).

Timing of noncardiac surgery after coronary revascularization

A delay is essential following either PCI or CABG before it is safe to proceed to noncardiac surgery.

Post percutaneous coronary intervention

PCI has evolved since balloon angioplasty was first introduced. Stents have greatly increased the proportion of lesions that can be safely tackled, providing a 'bail-out' option in the event of coronary dissection, and reducing the risk of later re-stenosis. A newer generation of drug-eluting stents is coated with a polymer impregnated with an anti-mitotic agent to prevent the proliferation of smooth muscle cells responsible for restenosis.

Until they become endothelialized, stents are vulnerable to subacute thrombosis, which carries a high mortality rate, and patients must be treated with aggressive antiplatelet medication, typically a combination of aspirin 75mg od with clopidogrel 75mg od. For bare-metal stents, 4–6 weeks of treatment before the clopidogrel can be discontinued is sufficient, though aspirin is continued indefinitely. Coated stents take longer to endothelialize, and the duration of combined treatment must therefore be longer, up to 1 year in some centres.

Noncardiac surgery performed early after PCI is hazardous, with a high risk of subacute stent thrombosis if combined antiplatelet therapy is withdrawn prematurely:

- bare-metal stents: risk 40–80% within 2 weeks of PCI; minimal after 6 weeks;
- drug-eluting stents: fewer data but danger period probably much longer;
- 'plain old balloon angioplasty' (POBA): cardiac event rate only 2% within 2 weeks; virtually nil thereafter.

The risk of significant postoperative haemorrhage on antiplatelet therapy is much lower than the risk of subacute stent thrombosis off it (7% versus 30% in one study).

Suggested approach to patients with PCI prior to noncardiac surgery

- POBA ideal; bare-metal stenting if necessary; avoid drug-eluting stents if at all possible.
- Delay surgery 2–4 weeks after POBA, 6 weeks after bare-metal stenting, or 6–12 months after drug-eluting stenting (until combined antiplatelet therapy discontinued).
- If noncardiac surgery essential within high-risk period, discuss with interventional cardiologist: probably safest to continue antiplatelet medication.

Post coronary artery bypass grafting

Patients undergoing vascular surgery within 1 month of CABG are at high risk (mortality 21% versus 4% in matched controls in one study). Surgery should be delayed for at least 6 weeks if at all possible.

Some have advocated combining CABG and peripheral vascular surgery (typically carotid endarterectomy) as a single procedure, but there is no convincing difference in overall outcome compared with separate operations performed in either order.

Beta-blockade

The majority of intermediate to high risk patients (≥ 3 Eagle criteria, with inducible ischaemia $\leq 25\%$ of the left ventricular myocardium) can undergo noncardiac surgery at acceptable risk under cover of beta-blockade.

- Start beta-blocker orally several days or weeks prior to surgery.
- Titrate dose to achieve resting heart rate 50–60bpm if tolerated (e.g. bisoprolol 5–10mg od).
- Carefully maintain beta-blockade intraoperatively and postoperatively aiming for heart rate < 80bpm: if necessary, give NG or IV (e.g. metoprolol boluses or esmolol infusion) until patient eating and drinking.
- Consider how long beta-blocker should be continued postoperatively, whether for duration of inpatient stay, for 30 days, or indefinitely (given the likely high long-term risk).

Notes
- Evidence strongest in the intermediate risk group. The Dutch Echocardiographic Cardiac Risk Evaluation (DECREASE) study investigated 112 patients undergoing major peripheral vascular surgery, who had ≥ 1 Eagle criterion and ischaemia on stress echo. The patients were randomized to bisoprolol or placebo.
  - Bisoprolol reduced cardiac death or nonfatal MI within 30 days of surgery from 34% to 3%.[9]
- There was no evidence of protection in patients with very extensive ischaemia (> 25% of left ventricular myocardium).
  - These patients were excluded from the DECREASE study.
  - Subsequent retrospective registry data suggested beta-blockade not protective in this group (consider angiography).
- No evidence to support simply beta-blocking everyone to avoid inconvenience of preoperative risk assessment:
  - Retrospective analysis of 663,635 patients showed beta-blockade only beneficial if patient's revised cardiac risk index criteria ≥ 2.[10]
  - Compared with placebo, beta-blocker did not reduce mortality or cardiac events at 18 months in 921 randomized diabetics.[11]

Other drugs

Preoperative clinical assessment provides an important opportunity to target cardiac risk factors, and the benefits may be more immediate than conventionally thought. One example is that of statins. In a study 100 vascular surgical patients were given atorvastatin 20mg od or placebo for 30 days before surgery, then 15 days afterwards, irrespective of cholesterol level.[12]

• Cardiovascular events reduced by one-third at 6 months postoperatively, irrespective of intitial cholesterol level.
• Possible plaque-stabilizing effect, independent of cholesterol lowering.

Postoperative cardiac monitoring and care

From a cardiac standpoint, the management priorities following peripheral vascular surgery are to minimize cardiac stress and monitor closely for evidence of ischaemia or infarction. These aims are better achieved in a high-dependency area rather than on a general ward.

Reduction of cardiac stress

Cardiac stress with increased myocardial oxygen demand is an important precursor to postoperative MI and must be minimized:
- good analgesia;
- careful attention to fluid-balance;
- correction of anaemia where necessary;
- maintenance of beta-blockade postoperatively, if necessary NG or IV;
- continuation of antiplatelet medication following coronary stenting.

Monitoring for ischaemia or infarction

Postoperative MI carries a mortality rate of 30–50%, three to four times higher than that of spontaneous MI, but may be hard to diagnose clinically:
- often no chest pain;
- less specific symptoms of dyspnoea, confusion, or hypotension.

Routine surveillance with ECGs and measurement of serum markers of myocardial necrosis, particularly the sensitive and cardiospecific troponins I and T, is therefore valuable.

Electrocardiography

Most myocardial infarctions are preceded by periods of ECG ischaemia, e.g. new abnormalities are seen on an immediate postoperative ECG in up to 10% of patients, doubling the risk of subsequent cardiac complications.
- Record 12-lead ECG preoperatively, immediately postsurgery in the recovery room, and on postoperative days 1, 2, and 3.
- New ST depression or T-wave inversion are worrying features, and more common than classical ST-elevation.

Serum troponins

The ability to assay serum troponins I and T has revolutionized the assessment of patients presenting to the emergency room with chest pain. Elevated levels identify patients at high risk of subsequent death or re-infarction. They are also of proven value in the postoperative setting (see Table 7.2).
- Measure troponin I or T (local preference) on postoperative days 1–3.
- Rise in troponin I to < 1.5ng/mL or T to < 0.1ng/mL:
  - modest risk;
  - conservative management initially;
  - consider further coronary investigation in outpatients.
- Rise in troponin I to ≥ 1.5ng/mL or T to ≥ 0.1ng/mL:
  - high postoperative mortality (23%);
  - discuss with cardiologist regarding early coronary angiography.

Table 7.2 Prognostic value of postoperative troponin I and T measurements in patients undergoing major peripheral vascular surgery

Ref.	N	Follow-up	Troponin ranges (ng/mL)	Patients	Mortality
13	229	6 months	I, ≤ 0.35	57%	5%
			I, 0.4–1.5	31%	7%
			I, 1.6–3.0	4%	20%
			I, > 3.0	8%	22%
14	447	2.7y	I, ≤ 0.6; T, ≤ 0.03	76%	13%
			I, 0.6–1.5; T, 0.03–0.1	15%	32%
			I, 1.5–3.1; T, 0.1–0.2	4%	25%
			I, > 3.1; T, > 0.2	5%	52%
15	393	4y	T, < 0.1		17%
			T, ≥ 0.1		41%
16	1152	In-patients	I, ≤ 0.2	85%	3%
			I, 0.2–1.4	10%	7%
			I, ≥ 1.5	5%	23%

Management of postoperative myocardial infarction

Despite careful preoperative assessment and optimal perioperative care, some patients undergoing peripheral vascular surgery will suffer MI in the postoperative period. Such patients have a high mortality rate and there are no randomized studies to guide their management, so this must be tailored to the individual. Management should be in a high dependency area, preferably the coronary care unit, with early and close involvement of an experienced cardiologist.

- Connect to ECG monitor and ensure defibrillator immediately available.
- Give 40% oxygen and ensure IV access.
- Perform rapid clinical assessment to clarify symptoms and identify pulmonary oedema or cardiogenic shock.
- Request chest radiograph.
- Give opiate analgesia for pain, whether cardiac or postoperative:
  - e.g. diamorphine 2.5–5mg IV with metoclopramide 10mg IV.
- Start aspirin if necessary:
  - e.g. 300mg orally or via nasogastric tube, then 75mg daily.
- Start or intensify beta-blockade if necessary and not contraindicated (e.g. by asthma, left ventricular failure, shock, or heart block), aiming for heart rate less than 70bpm:
  - e.g. metoprolol 5mg IV every 2min to maximum 15mg, then 50mg PO or NG after 15min, then 50mg qds; can be converted to once daily drug pre-discharge, e.g. bisoprolol 5–20mg.
- If postoperative haemostasis is secure, give sc low molecular weight heparin:
  - e.g. enoxaparin 100 units/kg bd.
- Give IV nitrate infusion for persistent chest pain:
  - e.g. glyceryl trinitrate 1–10mg/h, maintaining systolic blood pressure > 100mmHg.
- Give diuretic for left ventricular failure:
  - e.g. frusemide 80mg iv.

Further management depends on the clinical status and ECG appearances, and close liaison with an experienced cardiologist is mandatory.

- iv thrombolytic therapy is almost always *contraindicated* with the recent operation.
- Carefully consider immediate coronary angiography with a view to percutaneous intervention if ST elevation, or pulmonary oedema or cardiogenic shock, remembering that:
  - vascular access may be difficult;
  - severe multivessel coronary disease is likely but coronary artery bypass surgery is unattractive in the setting of postoperative MI;
  - intensive antiplatelet therapy is essential if coronary stenting performed.
- Patients with non-ST elevation MI who are clinically stable may be better managed conservatively in the first instance.

- If not already on them, consider adding:
  - statin (e.g. simvastatin 40mg PO od);
  - ACE-inhibitor (e.g. ramipril 2.5mg PO od, increasing gradually to 10mg over several days).
- If course uncomplicated, keep in hospital for at least 5–7 days
- If coronary angiography not performed as in-patient, ensure plan in place at discharge for outpatient angiography or noninvasive risk assessment, with early cardiology follow-up.

References

1 Hlatky MA, Boineau RE, Higginbotham MB, *et al.* (1989). A self-administered questionnaire to determine functional capacity (The Duke Activity Status Index). *Am J Cardiol* **64**, 651–4.

2 Fletcher GF, Balady G, Froelicher VF, *et al.* (1995). Exercise standards: a statement for health-care professionals from the American Heart Association. *Circulation* **91**, 580.

3 Lee TH, Marcantonio ER, Mangione CM, *et al.* (1999). Derivation and prospective validation of a simple index for prediction of cardiac risk of major noncardiac surgery. *Circulation* **100**, 1043–9.

4 L'Italien GJ, Paul SD, Hendel RC, *et al.* (1996). Development and validation of a Bayesian model for perioperative cardiac risk assessment in a cohort of 1,081 vascular surgical candidates. *J Am Coll Cardiol* **27**, 779–86.

5 Paul SD, Eagle KA, Kuntz KM, *et al.* (1996). Concordance of preoperative clinical risk with angiographic severity of coronary artery disease in patients undergoing vascular surgery. *Circulation* **94**, 1561–6.

6 Eagle KA, Rihal CS, Mickel MC, *et al.* (1997). Cardiac risk of noncardiac surgery: influence of coronary disease and type of surgery in 3368 operations. *Circulation* **96**, 1882–7.

7 Hassan SA, Hlatky MA, Boothroyd DB, *et al.* (2001). Outcomes of noncardiac surgery after coronary bypass surgery or coronary angioplasty in the Bypass Angioplasty Revascularization Investigation (BARI). *Am J Med* **110**, 260–6.

8 McFalls EO, Ward HB, Moritz TE, *et al.* (2004). Coronary-artery revascularization before elective major vascular surgery. *N Engl J Med* **351**, 2795–804.

9 Poldermans D, Boersma E, Bax JJ, *et al.* (1999). The effect of bisoprolol on perioperative mortality and myocardial infarction in high-risk patients undergoing vascular surgery. *N Engl J Med* **341**, 1789–94.

10 Lindenauer PK, Pekow P, Wang K, *et al.* (2005). Perioperative beta-blocker therapy and mortality after major noncardiac surgery. *N Engl J Med* **353**, 349–61.

11 DIPOM Trial Group (2006). Effect of perioperative beta blockade in patients with diabetes undergoing major non-cardiac surgery: randomised placebo controlled, blinded multicentre trial. *BMJ* **332**, 1482–5.

12 Durazzo AE, Machado FS, Ikeoka DT, *et al.* (2004). Reduction in cardiovascular events after vascular surgery with atorvastatin: a randomized trial. *J Vasc Surg* **39**, 967–75.

13 Kim LJ, Martinez EA, Faraday N, *et al.* (2002). Cardiac troponin I predicts short-term mortality in vascular surgery patients. *Circulation* **106**, 2366–71.

14 Landesberg G, Shatz V, Akopnik I, *et al.* (2003). Association of cardiac troponin, CK-MB, and postoperative myocardial ischemia with long-term survival after major vascular surgery. *J Am Coll Cardiol* **42**, 1547–54.

15 Kertai MD, Boersma E, Klein J, *et al.* (2004). Long-term prognostic value of asymptomatic cardiac troponin T elevations in patients after major vascular surgery. *Eur J Vasc Endovasc Surg* **28**, 59–66.

16 Le Manach Y, Perel A, Coriat P, *et al.* (2005). Early and delayed myocardial infarction after abdominal aortic surgery. *Anesthesiology* **105**, 885–91.

Anaesthesia for vascular surgery

General principles

- Anaesthesia for vascular surgery is a challenging subspeciality, requiring attentiveness and calmness under sometimes difficult circumstances. Vascular operations may be longer than predicted (by the surgeons, anyway!), and may involve large (sometimes sudden, unexpected, and unannounced) blood loss, with concomitant changes in haemodynamic variables.
- Vascular patients are usually elderly arteriopaths with significant associated diseases. Expect: hypertension; ischaemic heart disease (angina, MI); heart failure; diabetes mellitus; perhaps COPD (smoking). Poly-pharmacy is the rule—so again, expect: aspirin; a statin; a β blocker; diuretics; heart failure medications; and, perhaps, insulin/ oral hypoglycaemic agents.
- 30–40% of vascular operations are urgent, often out of hours. Anaes-thetic trainees may be the main anaesthetists for these patients. Some patients will already be anticoagulated; many others will receive anticoagulants perioperatively, so the choice of regional or general anaesthesia needs careful consideration. However, regional techniques can reduce morbidity and mortality (see below).
- All patients receiving synthetic grafts require antibiotic prophylaxis, which the anaesthetist should give before incision.
- Measure the blood pressure in both arms—there may be differences due to arteriopathy (use the higher of the two values clinically).
- All vascular patients require supplemental oxygen postoperatively for at least 24h to reduce the incidence of hypoxic episodes during the night.
- Vascular anaesthetists usually enjoy getting involved with the proce-dure. After all, they have chosen this speciality above many others! They particularly enjoy being informed of imminent large blood loss, aortic (carotid) clamping and unclamping.

Preoperative assessment

Clinical

The preoperative assessment is primarily directed at quantifying the extent of cardiorespiratory disease, in terms of the patient's ability to tolerate the physiological changes of the surgical procedure and post-operative period. Careful (documented) consideration should be given to the use of regional (epidural) anaesthesia. A careful history and examination should include direct questions about exercise tolerance (walking distance on the flat and ability to climb stairs) and the ability to lie supine.

Investigation

- FBC, U&E, clotting, ECG, CXR as appropriate.
- For aortic surgery and for patients with new, symptomatic cardiac disease, some dynamic assessment of cardiac function is required. This might include: stress echocardiography; radionuclide thallium scan; or, more fashionably, cardiopulmonary exercise testing. For some patients, coronary revascularization may be necessary before peripheral vascular surgery is attempted.
- Lung function tests may aid risk assessment in vascular surgical patients with COPD.

Premedication

Anxiolysis may be required for some. There is some evidence that β blockers given preoperatively may reduce cardiovascular mortality following major vascular surgery. This may even hold for a single dose of oral β blocker.

Management of the diabetic patient in the perioperative period

- Diabetic patients require special consideration and management in the perioperative period because surgery affects glycaemic control. Starvation and complex hormonal and metabolic changes in response to surgery cause a catabolic response due to an increase in sympathetic activity with release of glucagon and growth hormone. This results in gluconeogenesis, glycogenolysis, proteolysis, lipolysis, and ketogenesis. The effect is a state of hyperglycaemia and ketosis.
- Tight glycaemic control in the perioperative period has been shown to improve outcome and is thus the main aim in managing these patients. How this is achieved depends on the type of diabetes and the likely period of starvation.
- iv infusion of insulin, glucose, and potassium is now standard therapy and has replaced sc insulin therapy for the perioperative management of diabetes, especially in type 1 diabetic patients and patients with type 2 diabetes undergoing major procedures. Major surgery is defined as requiring GA of greater than 1h.
- Adequate fluids must be administered to maintain intravascular volume. Fluid deficits from osmotic diuresis in poorly controlled diabetes can be considerable. The preferred fluids are normal saline and dextrose saline. Fluids containing lactate (i.e. Ringer's lactate, Hartmann's solution) cause exacerbation of hyperglycaemia due to the rapid conversion of lactate to glucose.
- Two main methods of insulin delivery are used:
  - either combining insulin with glucose and potassium in the same bag (the GIK regimen); or
  - giving insulin separately with an infusion pump (sliding scale regimen).
- The combined GIK infusion is efficient, safe, and effective in many patients but does not permit selective adjustment of insulin delivery without changing the bag.
- The initial insulin infusion rate can be estimated as between one-half and three-quarters of the patient's total daily insulin dose expressed as units/h. Regular insulin, 1 unit/h, is an appropriate starting dose for most type 1 diabetic patients. Patients treated with oral antidiabetic agents who require perioperative insulin infusion, as well as insulin-treated type 2 diabetic patients, can be given an initial infusion rate of 1–2 units/h.
- Adequate glucose should be provided to prevent catabolism, starvation ketosis, and insulin-induced hypoglycaemia. The physiological amount of glucose required to prevent catabolism in an average nondiabetic adult is about 120g/day (or 5g/h). With preoperative fasting, surgical stress, and ongoing insulin therapy, the caloric requirement in most diabetic patients is 5–10g/h glucose. This can be given as 5 or 10% dextrose. An infusion rate of 100mL/h with 5% dextrose delivers 5g/h glucose. If fluid restriction is necessary, the more concentrated 10% dextrose can be used.

- The infusion of insulin and glucose induces an intracellular translocation of potassium, resulting in a risk for hypokalaemia. In patients with initially normal serum potassium, potassium chloride, 10mEq, should be added routinely to each 500mL of dextrose to maintain normokalaemia if renal function is normal.

Diet-controlled NIDDM

No special measures are required for minor surgery. With major surgery, monitoring blood glucose may detect a rise in blood sugar; this can be managed with boluses of short-acting insulin.

Oral hypoglycaemic controlled NIDDM

Minor surgery

Omit oral hypoglycaemic agent on the morning of surgery. Schedule surgery in the morning. Recommence therapy after first meal.

Major surgery

- Second-generation sulphonylureas should be discontinued 1 day before surgery, with the exception of chlorpropamide, which should be stopped 2 days before surgery. Other oral agents can be continued until the operative day.
- Although metformin has a short half-life of 6h, it is prudent to temporarily withhold therapy 1 day before surgery, especially in sick patients and those undergoing procedures that increase the risks for renal hypoperfusion, tissue hypoxia, and lactate accumulation. Patients treated with metformin should withhold the drug for 72h following surgery especially if iodinated radiocontrast has been used. Metformin therapy can be restarted after documentation of normal renal function and absence of contrast-induced nephropathy.
- Blood glucose levels need to be regularly monitored. If the sugars are high or starvation is to continue start an insulin regimen.

Insulin-dependent diabetes mellitus

- Ideally take the patent off long-acting insulins preoperatively and substitute short-acting insulin tds.
- Monitor blood sugar. On the morning of surgery start an infusion of an insulin regimen, e.g. 500mL 10% glucose, 10mmol potassium chloride, 10 units of insulin, and run at 1mL/kg/h. Continue this until feeding is established when the patient's normal regimen is re-introduced. The regimen may need adjusting and is titrated according to the blood sugar levels.

Regional anaesthesia in vascular surgical patients

Regional anaesthesia may be used alone for distal revascularization (epidural or spinal) and carotid endarterectomy (cervical plexus block). Supplemental sedation may be used to allay patient anxiety and reduce stress but is **no substitute** for adequate regional anaesthesia. Sciatic and femoral nerve blocks may be used to supplement general anaesthesia for distal revascularization. Epidural analgesia is commonly used to supplement general anaesthesia for AAA. The potential advantages of regional techniques in vascular surgical patients include:

- improved patient monitoring (CEA with awake patient);
- improved blood flow in legs, reduced DVT incidence, reduced re-operation rate (peripheral revascularization, amputation)—level 1 evidence;
- postoperative pain relief (AAA, distal revascularization);
- reduced pulmonary complications (AAA surgery)—level 1A evidence;
- pre-emptive analgesia for amputations—possible reduction in phantom limb pain—more controversial;
- treatment of proximal hypertension during aortic cross-clamp.

Note that epidural insertion will take up minutes of precious operating time and, on occasion, may take much longer. However, this is offset by your patients looking and feeling better, having less morbidity, and, even, mortality.

Contraindications to spinal/epidural analgesia

- Patient refusal (though they can often be persuaded!)
- Local sepsis (i.e. where the needle will be inserted) or bacteraemia—increased risk of epidural abscess.
- Bleeding diathesis—increased risk of epidural haematoma.
- True allergy to local anaesthetics (vanishingly rare).
- Fixed cardiac output conditions, e.g. aortic stenosis—the patient cannot increase the cardiac output in response to the systemic vasodilatation caused by spinal/epidural anaesthesia.

Epidurals and anticoagulation

The small but finite risk of epidural haematoma should be weighed up against the benefits of regional anaesthesia for each patient. As a general guide, epidural insertion (or post-op removal) should not be performed:

- in patients taking coumarin anticoagulants with INR > 1.5;
- in other coagulopathic patients, e.g. platelet count < 100×10^9/L;
- in patients who have received thrombolysis in the last 24h (urokinase/streptokinase);
- within 4h of minihep administration;
- within 12h of LMWH administration;
- within 2h of systemic heparinization;
- in patients receiving 'cardiac' heparin doses (e.g. 20,000 units).

Anaesthesia for abdominal aortic aneurysm (AAA) repair

Preoperative

- Elderly, often multiple co-morbidity. The mortality for elective aortic surgery is 5–10% (about 50:50, perioperative MI:multiorgan failure).
- Careful preoperative assessment. The ECG needs scrutinizing for signs of ischaemia. Check for renal impairment. A dynamic assessment of left ventricular function is required preoperatively.
- HDU/ICU for postoperative care. Pre-optimization is performed in some units—patients are admitted to the HDU/ICU a few hours pre-operatively to have lines, etc. inserted and to have haemodynamic status 'optimized'. This is controversial (and expensive).
- The usual cardiac medications should be continued, with a β-blocker added (e.g. atenolol 25mg) unless there is a good reason not to, e.g. reversible obstructive airway disease.

Perioperative

- Draw up vasoconstrictors (ephedrine and metaraminol) and have vasodilators (GTN) and beta-blockers (esmolol, labetalol) available.
- Minimum 2 × 14G or greater IV access. A hot air warmer and fluid warmer are essential.
- A Level-1® fluid warmer or equivalent is very useful for complex cases/redo/suprarenal clamp—they can bleed rapidly due to surgical problems/acidosis. Cell salvage is indicated if blood loss is > 1000mL.
- Arterial line and thoracic epidural (T6–T11) pre-induction. Take a baseline blood gas sometime before aortic cross-clamping.
- Use 5-lead ECG (leads II and V5)—this increases the sensitivity for detection of myocardial ischaemia up to 95%.
- Triple or quad lumen CVP after induction. Consider inserting a PA introducer as this will allow rapid fluid administration and facilitates PA catheter insertion if necessary. Continuous cardiac output monitoring, e.g. oesophageal Doppler, is useful during the cross-clamp period.
- Isovolaemic haemodilution pre-induction may be useful. AAA is ideal for this as you can return the patient's blood (with platelets and clotting factors) as the cross-clamp is coming off. As a rough guide: Hb = 10–12g/dL take 1 unit; Hb = 12–14g/dL take 2 units; Hb = 14–16g/dL take 3 units.
- Careful anaesthetic induction with monitoring of invasive arterial blood pressure. Use moderate/high-dose opioid, e.g. remifentanil (not worthwhile unless used with an epidural) or high-dose fentanyl (5–10mcg/kg). Treat hypotension with fluids at first and then, cautiously, vasoconstriction. Insert a urinary catheter for hourly measurement of urine output.
- Hypothermia is inevitable unless strenuous efforts are made to maintain temperature, particularly during induction and line insertion. Monitor core temperature. Do not place warming blankets on the lower limbs whilst the aorta is cross-clamped as this may worsen lower limb ischaemia.

- Heparin will need to be given just before cross-clamp. 3000–5000 units is usual. This may be reversed after unclamping with protamine 0.5–1mg/100 units heparin IV slowly—causes hypotension if given too fast.
- Proximal hypertension may follow aortic cross-clamping and is due to a sudden increase in SVR, increased SVC flow, and sympathoadrenal response. Treat by deepening anaesthesia ± beta-blocker (labetalol 5–10mg) ± GTN infusion.
- Whilst the aorta is clamped, metabolic acidosis will develop due to ischaemic lower limbs. Check arterial blood gases to assess haematocrit, metabolic acidosis, respiratory compensation, and ionized calcium.
- During the cross-clamp time (30–90min), start giving fluid, aiming for a moderately increased CVP, e.g. 5mmHg greater than at the start of the case by the time unclamping occurs. This helps with cardiovascular stability, reduces sudden hypotension following cross-clamp removal, and may help preserve renal function. Release of the cross-clamp by your helpful, friendly surgeon one limb at a time helps with haemodynamic stability.
- Hypotension following aortic unclamping is caused by a fall in SVR, relative hypovolaemia, and myocardial 'stunning' due to return of cold metabolic waste products from the legs, etc. Treat with:
  - IV fluids;
  - lightening anaesthetic depth;
  - boluses of adrenaline 10mcg aliquots (1mL of 1:100,000);
  - a bolus of calcium gluconate (up to 10mL 10%).
- Give isotonic crystalloid/colloid to replace insensible losses, 3rd space losses, and initial blood loss. Give blood products when a deficiency is identified, e.g. when haematocrit < 25% give blood, and when platelets < 100 × /L) give platelets. Check the activated clotting time (normal < 140sec) if you suspect coagulopathy. Thromboelastography will give you the whole coagulation picture. Protamine or aprotinin are worth considering for ongoing bleeding.

Postoperative

- ICU/HDU is essential postoperatively. HDU is appropriate for otherwise fit patients who are extubated at the end of the case. Extubate if warm, haemodynamically stable, and with a working epidural.
- Opioid infusion ± PCA if no epidural.
- Routine observations including invasive arterial and central venous pressure monitoring and urine output should be continued postoperatively to assess haemodynamic stability. There is a potential for large fluid shifts that will need replacement.

Special considerations

- Epidural diamorphine 2.5mg at induction will last for 12–24h. Use epidural LA sparingly until the aorta is closed—it is easier to treat aortic unclamping hypotension with a functioning sympathetic nervous system.

- Renal failure occurs in 1–2% but the mortality is 50% in those who develop it after AAA surgery. The position (suprarenal) and duration of cross-clamp time are the most important factors causing renal failure. Dopamine does not prevent renal failure, merely acting as an inotrope to increase GFR. Mannitol is used routinely by some (0.5g/kg during cross-clamp time) as it is a free-radical scavenger and an osmotic diuretic. The bottom line is: (a) work with a fast surgeon; (b) avoid hypovolaemia; and (c) monitor urine output hourly.

Anaesthesia for endovascular AAA repair

- Unless you are very fortunate, this will take place in the radiology suite—often far removed from the familiar theatre environment. Rapid blood loss and its consequences may be more difficult to manage here than in your familiar operating theatre—so expect the worst.
- Put large bore IV arterial and central venous lines in as for an open repair. Have at least one trained assistant who can help you if things get very exciting.
- Epidural anaesthesia alone will be more than adequate for the groin incisions, although some anaesthestists choose the stability and airway control of general anaesthesia throughout.
- If things go well, it will be a quiet day. The actual procedure of deploying the stent does not cause too many problems. Inflating the balloon to pressurize the deployed stent can cause transient hypertension. However, if the aneurysm ruptures, the mortality is 50%. You will need all the help you can get. It may be better to 'scoop and run' the patient back to the operating theatres rather than continue resuscitation in that unfamiliar environment.

Anaesthesia for emergency AAA repair

This is a true anaesthetic and surgical emergency. AAAs may rupture acutely—in which case cardiovascular collapse is the commonest presentation. Death is likely unless the rupture is contained in the retroperitoneal space. Alternatively, the aneurysm can dissect along the arterial intima or can expand rapidly. In these cases, back pain with or without abdominal pain is the usual presentation. Prehospital mortality for ruptured AAA is said to be 50%, and 50% of those reaching hospital also do not survive. Management is as for elective AAA, with the following additional considerations.

- Where doubt exists (but *only if* haemodynamic stability as well), diagnosis is confirmed by ultrasound/CT scan.
- If hypovolaemic shock is present, resuscitate to a systolic pressure of 90mmHg until the aortic cross-clamp is applied. Avoid hypertension, coughing, and straining at all costs as these may precipitate a further bleed. Titrate IV morphine against the patient's pain.
- Minimum lines pre-induction are two 14G peripheral cannulas and (ideally) an arterial line. Use of the brachial artery may be necessary and sometimes an arterial 'cut down' is indicated. Central venous access can wait until after the cross-clamp is applied. If peripheral veins are too shut down, insert a PA catheter sheath into the right internal jugular vein.
- Epidural analgesia is rarely appropriate because of time constraints preoperatively and coagulopathy postoperatively.
- A urinary catheter should be placed before induction.
- Induction must be in the operating theatre, with the surgeons scrubbed, surgical preparation completed, drapes on, and blood available in theatre and checked. A rapid sequence induction will usually be required (full stomach). Suitable induction agents include: midazolam/remifentanil; etomidate; or ketamine. As soon as the endotracheal tube is confirmed as being in the trachea ($ETCO_2$), let the surgeons know they can start. Treat hypotension with IV fluids and small doses of vasopressors/inotropes.
- Hot air warming and at least one warmed IVI are essential (a Level-1® blood warmer is invaluable).
- Have both IV lines running maximally at induction. One assistant should be dedicated to managing the IV fluid and ensuring an uninterrupted supply of appropriate fluids.
- Hypothermia, renal impairment, blood loss, and coagulopathy are common perioperative problems. Hypothermia is a particular hazard as, even if surgery goes well, the patient will continue to bleed on the ICU. Platelet function is markedly reduced below 35°C. Whilst there is no place for routine administration of platelets and FFP, consider early use when they are needed.
- Do not attempt to extubate at the conclusion of surgery—a postoperative period of ventilation on the ICU is essential to allow correction of biochemical and haematological abnormalities.

Anaesthesia for thoraco-abdominal and suprarenal aortic aneurysm repair

Thoracic aneurysms of the ascending aorta require median sternotomy and cardiopulmonary bypass. Transverse aortic arch repairs often require hypothermic circulatory arrest as well.

Special considerations

As for infrarenal AAA repair, with the following considerations.

- The aneurysm can compress the trachea and distort the anatomy of the upper vasculature.
- ICU is essential for postoperative ventilation and stabilization.
- The aortic cross-clamp will be much higher than for a simple AAA. This means that the kidneys, liver, and splanchnic circulation will be ischaemic for the duration of the cross-clamp.
- Access to the thoracic aorta may require one-lung ventilation—thus a left-sided double lumen tube may be required.
- Proximal hypertension following cross-clamping is more pronounced. Use aggressive vasodilatation with GTN (infusion of 50mg/50mL run at 0–5mL/h) or esmolol (2.5g/50mL at 3–15mL/h).
- Hypotension following aortic unclamping is often severe, requiring inotropic support postoperatively—use adrenaline 1:10,000 starting at 5mL/h.
- Acidosis may be a particular problem due to the metabolic acidosis that develops during cross-clamping and an additional respiratory acidosis due to prolonged one-lung ventilation.
- Renal failure occurs in up to 25% of cases—principally related to the duration of cross-clamp. Monitor urine output, give mannitol 25g before cross-clamping, and maintain the circulating volume during the case.
- Spinal cord ischaemia leading to paralysis may develop. This is related to the duration of cross-clamping and occurs because a branch of the thoracic aorta (artery of Adamkiewicz) reinforces the blood supply of the cord. Techniques used for prevention (none are infallible) include:
  - CSF pressure measurement and drainage through a spinal drain;
  - spinal cord cooling through an epidural catheter;
  - intrathecal magnesium;
  - distal perfusion techniques;
  - cardiopulmonary bypass and deep hypothermic circulatory arrest.
  - Surgeons performing this surgery have their own preferred techniques.
- Fluid balance is as for infrarenal AAA, although blood loss will be more extreme, blood transfusion will almost certainly be required, and platelets and FFP are more commonly required. Thromboelastography is essential to monitor the coagulation picture.
- Patients require ventilation postoperatively until acidosis and hypothermia are corrected and the lungs are fully re-expanded.

Anaesthesia for axillo-bifemoral bypass

This is often a last-chance operation for patients with completely occluded aortic or iliac arteries. Some will already have had aortic surgery and have infected grafts. It is an extraperitoneal operation, so patients with severe cardiorespiratory disease who might be excluded from aortic surgery may tolerate it better. However, do not be misled—it is still a long operation that can involve significant blood loss, morbidity, and even mortality.

Preoperative

The usual comments about preoperative assessment of vascular patients apply. Try to obtain recent information about cardiac function. An echocardiograph can easily be done at the bedside.

Some of these patients will be very sick, either from their pre-existing cardiorespiratory disease or from having infected aortic grafts. Surgery may be their only hope of life, although equally it can also be a rapid road to their demise. Provided the patient understands this, the operation may be appropriate despite high risk. These are not cases for inexperienced trainees to do alone.

Perioperative

- GA with ETT and IPPV is appropriate. An arterial line and a large-gauge cannula are mandatory. CVP monitoring is optional.
- Heparin/protamine will be required at clamping/unclamping.

Postoperative

- Extubation at the end of surgery is usually possible, but a period of time on the HDU is recommended if at all possible.
- PCA for postoperative analgesia.

Anaesthesia for carotid endarterectomy (CEA)

General or regional anaesthetic techniques are used. Monitoring cerebral perfusion during carotid cross-clamping is an important but controversial area. Advocates of regional anaesthesia cite the advantages of having a conscious patient in whom neurological deficits are immediately detectable and treatable.

Under GA, cerebral perfusion may be estimated/monitored as follows:
- measurement of carotid artery stump pressure;
- EEG processing;
- somatosensory evoked potentials monitoring;
- transcranial Doppler of the middle cerebral artery;
- cerebral oximetry;
- near-infrared spectroscopy.

Preoperative
- Most elderly arteriopathic patients are hypertensive. Determine the normal BP from ward charts. Measure BP in both arms. Aim for 160/90.
- Document pre-existing neurological deficits so that new deficits may be more easily assessed.
- Draw up vasoconstrictors (e.g. ephedrine and metaraminol) and have vasodilators available (e.g. GTN, labetalol).
- Consider which cerebral monitoring techniques to use.
- Premedication: sedative/anxiolytic, particularly if using GA.

Perioperative
- 20G and 14G IV access plus an arterial line for BP measurement—in the contralateral arm out on an arm board. 5-lead ECG monitoring, SpO_2, and $ETCO_2$.
- Maintain BP within 20% of baseline. During cross-clamping, maintain BP at or above baseline with vasoconstrictors, if required, e.g. metaraminol 0.5mg boluses. Such intervention can reverse new neurological deficits.

General anaesthesia for CEA
- Careful IV induction. Blood pressure may be very labile during induction and intubation. Most anaesthetists use an endotracheal tube although the LMA has been used. Consider spraying the cords with lidocaine 10% metered spray. Secure the tube and check tube connections very carefully (the head is inaccessible during surgery).
- Remifentanil infusion combined with superficial cervical plexus block gives ideal conditions, with rapid awakening. Otherwise isoflurane/opioid technique. Maintain normocapnia.
- Extubate deep before excessive coughing develops (this can exacerbate a haematoma). Close CNS monitoring in recovery until fully awake.

The 'awake carotid'

- Cervical dermatomes C2–C4 may be blocked by deep ± superficial cervical plexus block (or cervical epidural—rarely in the UK).
- Patient preparation and communication are vital. A thorough explanation of the awake technique is invaluable—this can usefully be initiated by the surgeon at the outpatient visit.
- For the deep block, 3 × 5mL 0.5% bupivacaine at C2, 3, and 4 or a single injection of 15mL 0.5% bupivacaine at C3. For the superficial block, 10mL 0.5% bupivacaine injected along the posterior border of sternocleidomastoid. The deep block should be avoided in patients with respiratory impairment as they may not tolerate the unilateral diaphragmatic paralysis that can ensue.
- Ensure the patient's bladder is empty preoperatively. Give IV fluids to replace blood loss only—catheterizing a full bladder whilst the carotid is cross-clamped is tricky.
- Take the patient's pillow and replace it with a soft head ring. Put the pillow under their knees to reduce back pain. An L-bar angled over the patient's neck allows good access for both surgeon and anaesthetist.
- Sedation (e.g. target-controlled propofol infusion 0.5–1mcg/mL, remifentanil infusion 0.05–0.1mcg/kg/min) can be used during block placement and dissection. No sedation during carotid cross-clamping will allow continuous neurological assessment. Administer oxygen throughout.
- Despite an apparently perfect regional block, 50% or so of patients will require LA supplementation by the surgeon, usually around the carotid sheath, or if the carotid bifurcation is very high. Feelings of claustrophobia are also common and usually respond to reassurance from the anaesthetist and/or cool air from a patient warmer being blown over the patient's face. Sips of water are also comforting for the patient.
- Monitor the patient's speech, contralateral motor power, and cerebration very closely during the carotid cross-clamp period. Neurological deficit presents in three ways:
  - profound unconsciousness on cross-clamping;
  - subtle but immediate deficit, e.g. confusion, slurred speech, delay in answering questions;
  - deficit after a variable time—related to relative hypotension.

If neurological deficit develops, a shunt should be inserted by the surgeon immediately, although your considerable tact/skill is required to reassure the patient, maintaining the airway whilst the shunt is being inserted. Recovery should be rapid once the shunt is in place—if it is not, convert to GA. Pharmacological augmentation of blood pressure may improve cerebration by increasing the pressure gradient of collateral circulation across the circle of Willis. Alternatively, increasing the inspired oxygen concentration has also been shown to improve cerebral oxygenation. A small number (2.5%) will require conversion to GA.

Postoperative

- Careful observation in recovery for ≥ 2h is mandatory. HDU is optimal if available, particularly for patients who develop a neurological deficit.

- Airway oedema is common—in both GA and regional cases—
  presumably due to dissection close to the airway. Cervical haematoma
  additionally occurs in 5% of cases. These need very careful observation
  in recovery. Immediate re-exploration is required for developing
  airway obstruction due to haematoma.
- BP must be controlled postoperatively to prevent hypovolaemic stroke
  and hyperperfusion syndrome. Careful written instructions should be
  given to ward staff about BP management. An example is:
  - 'If systolic BP > 160mmHg, call house officer and consider giving
    labetalol 5–10mg boluses IV or a hydralazine infusion. If systolic
    BP < 100mmHg, give IV fluid 250mL stat. and call medical staff.'
- New CNS symptoms and signs require immediate surgical consultation.

Anaesthesia for peripheral revascularization surgery

Preoperative

- These procedures constitute a large proportion of elective vascular surgery. The duration of surgery is very unpredictable—overruns are not uncommon. Vascular surgeons rarely overestimate the time that such an operation will take.
- Pay attention to preoperative assessment of the cardiovascular system. However, this surgery is better tolerated than AAA surgery. A dynamic assessment of cardiac function is not usually necessary, although new developments, e.g. unstable angina, do require investigation.
- The choice between general and regional anaesthesia is up to the individual. There is some evidence that regional anaesthesia is associated with lower re-operation rates. Long operations (> 4h) may make pure regional techniques impractical, but they are still possible.

Perioperative

- IV access: ensure you have at least one large (14 or 16G) IV cannula with an infusion that runs freely.
- Use invasive BP monitoring for long cases (> 2h), if haemodynamic instability is expected or in sicker patients. Otherwise, standard monitoring with five-lead ECG. CVP monitoring is rarely (never?) necessary.
- Regional anaesthesia is an alternative to GA offering good operating conditions with excellent postoperative pain relief. Single-shot spinal anaesthesia alone may not give enough time for some procedures. The combination of spinal and epidural anaesthesia is ideal. If the patient can lie affected side down, hyperbaric bupivacaine (2–2.5mL 0.5%) can be used to produce a very dense spinal block on that side. Consider giving epidural diamorphine 1–2mg initially, then start an epidural infusion of 0.25% bupivacaine at 5–10mL/h after an hour or so. Always give supplemental oxygen. If the patient wants to be sedated, use the CO_2 sampling tubing within the oxygen face mask so that respiratory rate can be monitored as well.
- Heparin, e.g. 3000–5000 units, will need to be given before clamping. Reverse with protamine 0.5–1mg/100 units heparin slowly after unclamping if necessary.

Postoperative

- Epidural infusion. PCA if no epidural. Postoperative pain may even be less than the preoperative, ischaemic pain.
- Oxygen overnight.

Anaesthesia for amputations

Preoperative

- Commonly, sick, bed-bound diabetics with significant cardiovascular disease who have had repeated revascularization attempts previously.
- Many will be in considerable discomfort preoperatively (less so the diabetics due to the peripheral neuropathy) and may be on large doses of enteral or parenteral opioids. Regional analgesia may give more predictable results than parenteral opioids postoperatively.

Perioperative

- Spinal anaesthesia with hyperbaric bupivacaine and sedation offers excellent anaesthesia that can be directed affected side down. The duration of block (and postoperative pain relief) can be extended with intrathecal diamorphine (0.25–0.5mg) ± clonidine 15mcg intrathecally.
- Epidural analgesia offers better postoperative analgesia and can be sited preoperatively if required (pre-emptive analgesia).
- GA is also an option, but additional regional blockade is advisable (combined sciatic and femoral blocks will ensure analgesia for up to 24h).
- Occasionally these patients are septic due to the necrotic tissue. The only way they will get better is to have the affected part amputated. Thus the operation should *not* be cancelled for this reason.

Postoperative

- Regional analgesia is the best option; otherwise PCA.
- Phantom limb pain is a problem for 60–70% amputees at some time. It must be distinguished from surgical pain in the stump (which can be treated by conventional analgesic techniques). Phantom limb pain often requires chronic pain team input.
- Pre-emptive analgesia (i.e. siting and using the epidural preoperatively) is believed by some to reduce the incidence and severity of chronic pain. This is controversial.
- Combined sciatic/femoral nerve blocks are an alternative to an epidural, particularly when the patient is receiving anticoagulation.
- Even with perfect regional analgesia you may need to continue enteral opioids postoperatively

Anaesthesia for thoracoscopic sympathectomy

- Patients are usually young, fit people with hyperhidrosis (sweaty palms and axillae).
- Traditionally, this is done using one-lung anaesthesia (double lumen tube) with the patient in the reverse Trendelenburg position.
- A simpler technique involves the patient breathing spontaneously through an LMA. When the surgeon insufflates CO_2 into the pleural cavity, the lung is pushed away passively, allowing surgery to take place. The degree of shunt produced is less dramatic than with one-lung ventilation. Assisted ventilation must be avoided, except to re-inflate the lung manually at the end. The CO_2 insufflator machine regulates intrapleural pressures.
- With either technique, at the conclusion of the procedure, the lung must be re-expanded (under the surgeon's direct vision) to abolish the pneumothorax.
- Local anaesthetic can be deposited by the surgeon directly on to the sympathetic trunk and into the pleural cavity.
- A postoperative chest radiograph is required to confirm that the lung has re-inflated sufficiently.
- Synchronous bilateral sympathectomies are a much more challenging operation. This can lead to very profound hypoxia when the second lung is collapsed due to persistent atelectasis in the first lung. It is certainly inappropriate for all but the very fittest patients.

Further reading

Caldicott L, Lumb A, McCoy D (2000). *Vascular anaesthesia, a practical handbook.* Butterworth Heinemann, Oxford.

O'Connor CJ, Rothenburg DM (1995). Anesthetic considerations for descending thoracic aortic surgery: Parts 1 and 2. *J Cardiothorac Vasc Anesth* **9**, 581–8, 734–47.

Mukherjee D, Eagle KA (2003). Perioperative cardiac assessment for noncardiac surgery: eight steps to the best possible outcome. *Circulation* **107**, 2771–4.

Stoneham MD, Knighton JD (1999). Regional anaesthesia for carotid endarterectomy. *Br J Anaesth* **82**, 910–19.

Poldermans D, et al. (1999). The effect of bisoprolol on perioperative mortality and myocardial infarction in high-risk patients undergoing vascular surgery. *N Engl J Med* **341**, 1789–94.

Shine TS, Murray MJ (2004). Intraoperative management of aortic aneurysm surgery. *Anesthesiol Clin N Am* **22**, 289–305.

Lippmann M, et al. (2003). Anesthesia for endovascular repair of abdominal and thoracic aortic aneurysms: a review article. *J Cardiovasc Surg (Torino)* **44**, 443–51.

Christopherson R, et al. (1993). Perioperative morbidity in patients randomized to epidural or general anesthesia for lower extremity vascular surgery. Perioperative Ischemia Randomized Anesthesia Trial Study Group 1993. *Anesthesiology* **79**, 422–34.

Chapter 9

Managing coagulation and bleeding

Perioperative coagulation

In the patient undergoing vascular surgery, coagulation must be sufficiently effective to ensure haemostasis despite vascular anastomoses and often extensive dissection. Set against this is the need for adequate antico-agulation to prevent clot formation on thrombogenic surfaces (such as endarterectomized arteries or prosthetic graft materials) or thrombosis of relatively static blood in clamped vessels. These goals can be achieved by careful assessment and correction of coagulation perioperatively, and by the use of local and systemic anticoagulants and their antagonists during surgery.

Preoperative assessment and correction

All patients undergoing any form of vascular surgery should have an assessment of their coagulation status preoperatively. This should include the following.

- Drug history.
  - Use of anti-platelet drugs, e.g. aspirin, clopidogrel, or dipyridamole. Surgery can safely be carried out in the presence of a single agent. If two are being taken in combination, one should be stopped 1 week prior to surgery. The continued use of clopidogrel may preclude epidural anaesthesia because of the risk of epidural haematoma.
  - Patients on oral anticoagulants, usually warfarin, will need to stop them preoperatively. Patients taking anticoagulants for atrial fibrillation or previous thromboembolic events should be instructed to stop them 5 days preoperatively. They should be admitted on the day prior to surgery to check the international normalized ratio (INR) to ensure that the effect of the anticoagulant has dissipated. These patients should receive standard perioperative thromboem-bolic prophylaxis with low molecular weight heparin (LMWH).
  - Patients with prosthetic heart valves will need systemic anticoagula-tion with IV unfractionated or SC LMWH while the effects of warfarin wear off. This can either be done as an inpatient or as an outpatient with daily SC LMWH administered by district nurses, if local facilities allow. If using unfractionated heparin, the target activated partial prothrombin time (APTT) is 1.5–2.5× normal.
- Past history or family history of thrombosis.
  - A strong past or family history of arterial or venous thrombo-embolic disease raises the possibility of a thrombophilic tendency, such as protein S and protein C deficiency, anti-phospholipid syndrome, or factor V Leiden.
  - It should also be suspected in unusually young patients presenting with vascular disease.
  - If thrombophilia is suspected, perform a thrombophilia screen (factor V Leiden, protein C and S, antithrombin, lupus anticoagulant) and obtain haematologist's advice if positive result. Confirmation of the diagnosis may indicate the need for more aggressive anticoagulation therapy perioperatively.
- History of bleeding tendencies.

- If there is a history of bleeding tendencies, such as factor VIII deficiency or von Willebrand's disease, ensure that a supply of the relevant factor is available at the time of surgery.
- History of malignancy.
  - The presence of malignant disease may render the patient hypercoagulable, perhaps requiring more aggressive anticoagulant therapy, although the risks of bleeding from the tumour itself must be remembered.
- Blood tests.
  - FBC. A platelet count of $< 50 \times 10^9$/L is likely to result in impaired coagulation. A count $> 400 \times 10^9$/L may be associated with increased tendency to thrombosis.
  - INR and APTT. Ratios of greater than 2 times control should be corrected prior to surgery, unless systemic anticoagulation is indicated, as above.
- Correction of clotting abnormalities.
  - A low platelet count should be corrected with platelet transfusion at induction, on advice from a haematologist.
  - If the INR is elevated secondary to oral anticoagulation, elective surgery should be deferred until it has normalized.
  - Where urgent surgery needs to be carried out or if the elevated INR is secondary to other factors, e.g. liver disease, 5mg of vitamin K should be administered po or iv. This will, however, delay re-establishment of oral anticoagulation postoperatively.
  - If emergency surgery is indicated, anticoagulation can be reversed using fresh frozen plasma (FFP). The number of units required will depend on the INR.
  - In patients receiving an iv infusion of unfractionated heparin preoperatively, cessation 4 hours prior to surgery should allow the APTT to fall to acceptable levels for surgery.

Intraoperative anticoagulation

- After exposure of the vessels being operated on and completion of any other major dissection required (such as formation of tunnels for grafts), systemic anticoagulation is achieved by administration of iv unfractionated heparin. A dose of 5000 IU will suffice in patients of average build but should be adjusted for those with larger or smaller frames (70u/kg). Heparin given in this way has a half-life of 30–240min. A repeat dose may be required for long procedures.
- A solution of 5000 IU heparin in 1L of normal saline (5IU/mL) is used during surgery. This can be instilled into vessels prior to clamping to reduce the risk of thrombosis. It is also useful to fill grafts with this solution when they have to be clamped having been perfused. Irrigation of luminal or endarterectomized surfaces during surgery aids vision and reduces clot formation.
- Where reversal of systemic heparinization is required at the end of the procedure, protamine can be given iv. One mg neutralizes 80–100IU of heparin when given within 15min, but less is required if the delay is longer. In overdose, protamine has anticoagulant activity. Protamine given too quickly iv can cause hypotension.

- In addition to standard tests of anticoagulation, such as INR and APTT, thromboelastography (TEG) may be used to monitor coagulation intraoperatively. TEG is a global test of blood clotting that can be rapidly performed in the operating theatre. The results can be used to guide intraoperative anticoagulation and its reversal.

Control of intraoperative haemorrhage

A number of factors other than anticoagulant drugs may impair coagulation in patients undergoing major vascular surgery.

- Hypothermia may severely impair coagulation. This can be minimized by keeping the operating theatre warm, limiting exposure of the patient, using hot air warming blankets, administration of warmed IV fluids, and minimizing loss of heat from exposed bowel by wrapping in packs and a bowel bag.
- Massive transfusion of autologous blood (> 10 units) may result in a profound coagulopathy.

Management of haemorrhage

- Maximize warming of the patient.
- In the presence of massive transfusion, administer FFP and platelets. These should not be given until all clamps have been removed. These products may take some time to procure, so their requirement should be anticipated by the clinical scenario, such as a ruptured aneurysm.
- Reverse the effects of systemic heparin (see 'Intraoperative coagulation', p. 159).
- Aprotinin (Trasylol®) is of maximum benefit in hyperfibrinolytic haemorrhage such as is seen in extracorporeal circulation. However, it may be of benefit in coagulopathic vascular patients. An initial dose of 500,000kIU can be supplemented by 200,000kIU every 4h up to a maximum of 7,000,000kIU.
- The use of recombinant activated factor VII (rfFVIIa) has been described as a salvage treatment in severe haemorrhage from a number of causes, including disseminated intravascular coagulation, the action of fibrinolytic agents, massive transfusion, and hypothermia, with promising results. A single bolus IV dose of 90mcg/kg is given. Recombinant factor VII is very expensive.
- For local control of haemorrhage, such as at an anastomosis, simple pressure (and time) may be augmented by use of alginate materials with high calcium contents that promote coagulation locally. Some of these are absorbable and may be left in situ. Fibrin glues can also be applied to suture lines, but require the area to be dry during application.
- In the cold, coagulopathic patient at the end of major abdominal vascular surgery, packing of the abdomen is sometimes the last resort for control of haemorrhage. Under these circumstances, the patient's abdomen should be closed over packs prior to transfer to the ICU. There, the patient can be warmed and coagulation optimized, prior to removal of packs the next day.

Postoperative anticoagulation

- For the majority of patients, standard thromboembolic prophylaxis with LMWH, together with their usual antiplatelet drug, is adequate postoperative anticoagulation.
- Antiplatelet therapy will reduce the incidence of cardiac events in patients with arterial disease, but has no benefit with regard to patency rates of short vein grafts. However, antiplatelet drugs will improve the patency of prosthetic femoro-popliteal grafts.
- In patients with grafts felt to be at high risk of occlusion (those in whom grafts have previously occluded, those with very long grafts, those with poor run-off or suboptimal conduit), the use of systemic anticoagulation will improve primary patency. The patient should be heparinized at the end of surgery and oral anticoagulation begun the next day, provided there is no sign of postoperative haemorrhage. Aim for a target INR of 2–2.5.
- It is unclear how long anticoagulation should be continued in high-risk revascularizations. Where large areas of endarterectomized vessel are present, discontinuation may be considered after a few weeks when a neo-intima will be fully formed. For high-risk bypass grafts, it should probably be continued for the life of the graft.

Heparin-induced thrombocytopenia (HIT)

In up to 3% of patients treated with unfractionated heparin (and about 0.1% of those receiving LMWH) a fall in platelet count is observed. This is due to heparin-induced platelet antibodies, which may result in life-threatening thrombosis. Onset is 4 days to 2 weeks after treatment begins. Two types of HIT are described.

Type 1

- Characterized by transient fall in platelet count, though rarely below 100×10^9/L. Usually recovers spontaneously, even if heparin continued.
- Does not usually result in life-threatening thrombosis.
- Heparin should be discontinued.
- Anticoagulation with warfarin may be instituted if indicated.

Type 2

- Platelet count often falls to $< 60 \times 10^9$/L.
- Results from combination of heparin with platelet factor 4, with subsequent clumping of platelets.
- May be associated with life-threatening thrombosis.
- Skin necrosis may occur at infusion site.
- Protamine and warfarin are ineffective.
- Treatment is with danaparoid, lepirudin, bivalirudin, or argatroban.

Thrombolysis

Catheter-directed infusion of thrombolytic agents can be used to dissolve recent thrombus, as primary therapy in the treatment of acute limb ischaemia and venous thrombosis. It also has a role as an adjunct to surgery for ischaemic limbs (on-table thrombolysis).

Alteplase (recombinant tissue plasminogen activator, rt-PA) is the preferred thrombolytic agent. It acts by converting plasminogen to plasmin, which degrades fibrin, so breaking up thrombus. It is metabolized principally in the liver and has a half-life of 5min. Unlike streptokinase, rt-PA does not carry the risk of sensitivity reactions. The major hazard associated with thrombolysis is haemorrhage.

Contraindications to thrombolysis

- Recent haemorrhage, trauma, or surgery (3 months).
- Recent arterial puncture, e.g. for arteriography.
- Bleeding disorder or warfarin anticoagulation.
- History of stroke, CNS tumour, or spinal surgery.
- Severe uncontrolled hypertension.
- Haemorrhagic retinopathy.
- Neoplasm with increased bleeding risk.
- Liver disease or oesophageal varices.
- Pancreatitis or recent peptic ulcer.

Thrombolysis for acute lower limb ischaemia

Thrombolysis (± balloon angioplasty) can be used as an alternative to surgery for the treatment of acute limb ischaemia.

Thrombolysis should be considered when:

- there is a short duration of ischaemia (less than 2 weeks);
- there is distally placed thrombus (less risk of distal embolization);
- there is a low risk of compartment syndrome (fasciotomies not required);
- the patient has normal renal function (large doses of contrast medium may be needed).

Preparation

- Arrange nursing with close observation in a high dependency setting to monitor for bleeding complications.
- Cross-match 4 units of blood.
- Commence a low dose heparin infusion (500IU/h) to prevent further propagation of thrombus.
- Duplex scan may be useful in planning approach to thrombolysis.

Procedure

- Obtain a percutaneous transfemoral angiogram and direct a catheter into the thrombus under angiographic guidance.
- Inject a 5mg bolus of rt-PA into the thrombus.
- Infuse rt-PA at a dose of 1mg/h over 4 hours.
- Repeat angiography after infusion is completed.

- Repeat cycles of 4h infusion and angiography until:
  - there is resolution of the thrombus;
  - there is no difference between subsequent angiograms; or
  - a complication occurs.
- Consider adjunctive radiological procedures including angioplasty and stenting at check angiography.
- Thrombus resolution should be achieved within 24h. The risks of thrombolysis increase considerably after this time.

Management of bleeding associated with thrombolysis

- Stop infusion
- Compress bleeding point
- Resuscitate as required
- Check fibrinogen, PT, APTT, and FBC
- Consider giving aprotinin (500,000 units over 5min) and clotting factors as required

On-table thrombolysis for arterial occlusion

Catheter-directed thrombolysis might be employed as an adjunct or alternative to embolectomy in cases of recent in situ thrombosis or distal embolization including trash foot. It may be particularly useful in thrombus affecting distal small vessels, for acute on chronic disease or for delayed presentation (1–2 weeks) of acute limb ischaemia.

Preparation and procedure

- First perform standard balloon embolectomy.
- Flush with heparinized saline.
- Perform on-table angiogram to establish site of distal thromboembolic occlusion.
- Infuse a 5mg bolus of rt-PA through the catheter.
- Infuse a further 15mg over 20min.
- Check angiogram.
- Consider repeating if there is partial resolution.

Thrombolysis for deep venous thrombosis (DVT)

The use of thrombolysis for DVT is generally reserved for ilio-femoral DVT associated with gross oedema or cases of phlegmasia caerulea dolens.

Its use in these cases may resolve symptoms and is associated with an improvement in long-term venous function. It may also be given through an intra-arterial catheter. Adjunctive procedures, including venous stenting and filter placement, may be employed.

Procedure
- Insert catheter through the femoral artery, femoral vein, or popliteal vein.
- Infuse 1mg rt-PA/h.
- Give heparin IV infusion at 500IU/h.
- Check coagulation screen every 4h and adjust heparin to keep APTT between 40 and 60sec.
- Check venogram after 8h.
- Continue cycles for up to 24h.

Minimizing transfusion requirements in vascular surgery

- Jehovah's Witnesses believe that blood should not be removed from the body and stored. They will not accept transfusion of whole blood or its components, i.e. red blood cells, white blood cells, platelets, or plasma. The use of more highly fractionated components of blood, such as clotting factors or interferons, is left to the individual.
- Increasing numbers of patients are now requesting the avoidance of blood transfusion for reasons other than religious belief. Principal among these is avoidance of transmission of blood-borne infections. All transfused blood is screened for serious pathogens such as the hepatitis viruses. However, there have been instances of infection with diseases before screening has been established or when screening is not possible, such as in HIV or prion diseases like new-variant Creutzfeldt–Jakob disease. Some patients are concerned about possible transfusion reactions because of medical error. A small number of cases continue to occur in the UK annually despite measures to minimize them (439 cases reported in 2004).
- Patients who have received multiple blood transfusions in the past can be difficult to cross-match because of large numbers of atypical antibodies.
- Blood transfusion is expensive. Provision of blood and blood products for transfusion in the UK cost close to 1 billion pounds in 2000–2001.
- The availability of blood also continues to decline as the population ages, since elderly people consume more blood products than they donate. Some vascular operations (such as carotid endarterectomy and elective aneurysm repair) are essentially prophylactic procedures. Others, such as surgery for intermittent claudication, are treating lifestyle limiting rather than life-threatening conditions. Under these circumstances, the inability to transfuse may alter the risk–benefit ratio such that conservative management is preferred.
- For those who require surgery, strategies have been developed to avoid major blood transfusion.

Preoperative preparation

- Pre-existing anaemia must be identified and any treatable cause addressed. The patient should be screened for disorders of clotting, including any family history of bleeding diatheses.
- Optimization of preoperative haemoglobin concentration may be achieved by a diet rich in iron, supplemented if necessary by iron, folate, and vitamin B_{12} supplements in the weeks prior to surgery. Vitamin C aids iron absorption from the gut.
- Bone marrow production of erythrocytes can be increased by treatment with erythropoietin (EPO) in the weeks prior to surgery. Patients can be given recombinant human erythropoietin (rHuEPO) at 300 units/kg daily for 4 days or 300–600 units/kg weekly for 3 weeks prior to surgery. Production of leucocytes and platelets may be stimulated by the administration of GM-CSF and IL-11, respectively.

- Smoking cessation prior to surgery will maximize the oxygen-carrying capacity of the available haemoglobin.
- Minimization of number and volume of preoperative blood tests, including the use of microanalysers that require much smaller quantities of blood.
- Patients who wish to avoid transfusion with blood products should be clearly identified with the use of a distinctive wristband identifier. Their notes and drug and fluid charts should be prominently marked with appropriate stickers. Patients should sign a specific consent form or advance directive that confirms their refusal of blood products after a discussion of the consequences of non-transfusion.

Intraoperative strategies

Anaesthetic techniques

- The use of 100% inspired oxygen during surgery maximizes oxygen carriage of the blood.
- Hypotensive anaesthesia maintains the blood pressure at the minimum level required to maintain adequate perfusion of essential organs, thus minimizing any bleeding that occurs. This may be precluded by the coexistence of coronary arterial disease or haemodynamically significant carotid stenoses.
- Hypothermia should be avoided as blood clotting is impaired under these circumstances.
- Fluid losses during surgery can be replaced using colloid and/or crystalloid fluids. Perfluorocarbon solutions supplement oxygen-carrying capacity in addition to volume expansion. Several acellular haemoglobin solutions, containing either recombinant human haemoglobin or polymerized bovine haemoglobin, have been the subject of clinical trials.
- Haemodilution during surgery reduces the red cell content of any blood lost. In normovolaemic haemodilution, blood is drawn off prior to fluid administration. At the end of the procedure, the withdrawn blood is returned to the patient. Some Jehovah's Witnesses find this technique acceptable, providing the blood has continued to circulate within a closed system throughout.
- Some patients may also accept use of cell salvage systems that recover and concentrate red cells removed from the operative field by suction, provided that a closed system is used. Such systems cannot be used in patients with malignancy or on-going sepsis.

Surgical techniques

- Meticulous attention to haemostasis by immediate ligation or coagulation of any bleeding vessels during surgery will reduce intraoperative blood loss.
- Use of pharmacological agents to reduce bleeding, such as transexamic acid or activated factor VII.

- Novel surgical instruments may also help to minimize blood loss during open surgery, though the evidence for this is currently sparse.
  - Argon gas beam coagulators are claimed to achieve haemostasis more rapidly and efficiently than conventional radiofrequency electrocautery.
  - Harmonic scalpels have a tip that vibrates at ultrasonic frequencies and denatures and divides tissue with minimal heat generation, allowing simultaneous cutting and coagulation.

Postoperative strategies

Until relatively recently, patients were normally transfused if their Hb concentration fell below 10g/dL or their haematocrit below 0.30. However studies in critical care have not demonstrated any adverse effect from transfusing patients only when the Hb falls below 7g/dL. The use of a lower trigger for giving blood will obviate the need for transfusion in many postoperative patients. The exception to this policy is the patient with coronary arterial disease in whom anaemia may provoke myocardial ischaemia.

Minimally invasive and endovascular techniques

- Interventional radiological techniques may be considered as an alternative to open surgery. Aorto-iliac stenoses or short occlusions can often be treated by transluminal balloon angioplasty, with placement of a stent if the lesion is recurrent or persists after angioplasty. Treatment of long occlusions (greater than 10cm in length) in the superficial femoral or popliteal arteries has previously required femoro-popliteal bypass surgery. The advent of subintimal balloon angioplasty has allowed the interventional radiological treatment of such lesions. Some proponents of this technique have been able to achieve good results from angioplasty of lesions that would normally require femoro-distal bypasses, sometimes even to the ankle. The long-term durability of this technique, particularly for long lesions, remains unclear.
- Successful laparoscopically-assisted and totally laparoscopic AAA repair and ilio-femoral bypass have been reported. These procedures can be carried out through much smaller incisions than in conventional open surgery, with a possible reduction in blood loss. However, to date, no randomized controlled studies have been conducted to prove this.
- Randomized controlled trials have demonstrated reduced blood loss and transfusion requirements in endovascular repair of thoracic and abdominal aortic when compared to conventional open repair.

Legal considerations

- It is illegal to give blood or blood products to a competent adult against their wishes, even when it is considered to be life-saving.
- In unconscious or otherwise incompetent adults, the situation is less clear. Many Jehovah's Witnesses carry advance directive cards that make their refusal of blood products explicit or have given a copy of an advance directive to friends or relatives. The production of such documents prevents clinicians from being held liable for the results if transfusion is withheld. Treatment with blood products in the face of

evidence of the patient's wishes is probably unlawful. However, the exact legal status of advance directives in England and Wales remains unclear and no Act of Parliament has been passed concerning them. If the patient is not able to articulate their wishes and no documentary evidence can be produced, then the doctor's clinical judgement takes precedence. Such scenarios are only likely to be encountered in emergency situations but may be relevant in aneurysmal rupture, for example, where patients are often obtunded. In this situation, survival would be unlikely without transfusion.

- The situation is even more complex in children, although major vascular surgery is rarely required other than in trauma. In England and Wales, children of 16 and 17 years are deemed competent to give consent, even if this is against the wishes of their guardians. Children younger than this can also give consent if it is felt they understand the procedure. However, a child under 16 cannot refuse a treatment if their guardians consent to it. Thus, older children of Jehovah's Witnesses may consent to receive blood products against the wishes of their parents. If, after full consultation, parents refuse permission for transfusion, then the surgeon in England and Wales can seek a Specific Issue Order from the courts to protect the child's best interests. This provides legal authority for administration of blood for a specific condition.
- Where doubt remains about the appropriate action on legal or ethical grounds, advice should be sought from in-hospital legal services and medical defence bodies.

Useful contacts/further information

Jehovah's Witnesses Hospital Liaison Committees can assist with management of Jehovah's Witness patients and can also provide specialized consent forms. Hospital Information Services: 020 8906 2211.

The official website of the Jehovah's Witnesses organization provides a summary of their beliefs with regard to blood and blood products, as well as numerous links to related medical sites. www.watchtower.org

Infection prophylaxis and treatment

Introduction

The healthy body supports a large number of indigenous organisms. These organisms coexist with the host and do not normally cause disease. The body has a number of defence mechanisms against the establishment of pathogenic organisms. The process of diseases and/or surgical treatments can compromise these defences such that microbiological organisms can cause clinical infection.

The hospital environment

Merely being admitted to hospital exposes patients to organisms that they would not normally encounter in their everyday life. Species such as methicillin-resistant *Staphylococcus aureus* (MRSA) and pseudomonads are prevalent in the hospital environment and are readily transmissible to new patients mainly by skin to skin contact from health care workers. A patient on antibiotics is at additional risk as their normal flora is reduced and resistant organisms can easily become established. Special areas such as HDUs or ICUs harbour unusual and idiosyncratic organisms, often as a consequence of the use of broad spectrum antibiotics in patients for prolonged periods of time.

The immunocompromised patient

Patients with rare inherited forms of immunodeficiency, HIV infection, and asplenism and elderly or diabetic patients are especially susceptible to infection. Drugs such as steroids are immunosuppressant and transplant recipients take intentionally immunosuppressant medication. This will usually be apparent from the history and precautions can be taken.

Portals of entry

Surgery necessarily involves the loss of the integrity of the skin and may involve entry into various body cavities. Major vascular surgery involves the use of endotracheal tubes, monitoring lines, and catheters further compromising physical barriers to infection. Each breach is a potential portal of entry, which may cause a bacteraemia potentially giving access to infection at any distant site. Clinicians need to adhere to strict aseptic technique to reduce the risk of contamination.

Clean skin wounds

The most common organism implicated is *Staphylococcus aureus*. This can be seeded into the wound from an exogenous source, e.g. from skin scales of a carrying member of the team falling into the wound, or from an endogenous source, the patient themselves. Approximately 20% of people have *S. aureus* as part of their skin or nasal flora. However, the majority of these are not pathogenic strains and it is not helpful to identify carriers. A more common source is active dispersal from a suppurating skin infection either from the patient or staff. The lesion in the patient should be covered with an occlusive dressing. Staff with a boil or caruncle should not be allowed into the operating theatre until it is healed. Other high dispersers are staff with severe eczema or groin fungal infections.

In the event of an outbreak of surgical site infection the specific strain of organism can be identified and traced. The GI tract is not intentionally breached in vascular surgical operations and the peritoneum should remain sterile. The sort of organisms found in surgical site infections after bowel surgery (*Escherichia coli*, *Enterobacter*, *Klebsiella*, *Enterococcus*) should not occur after vascular surgery.

Prophylactic antibiotics

- Prophylactic antibiotics have been shown to reduce surgical site infection. They should be administered so they have maximum and adequate concentration just prior to the skin incision or the placement of lines for major surgery. They should not be continued after the end of surgery but, if the operation is prolonged, e.g. more than 4h, a further dose should be given during surgery depending on the half-life of the antibiotic.
- Local policy should dictate the particular choice and combination based on microbiological advice. The local conditions dictate the prevalence of pathogenic strains and resistance, as well as data on recent surgical site infections. For vascular surgery broad spectrum cover is given, e.g. cefuroxime 1.5g iv and metronidazole 500mg iv. Where prosthetic grafts are employed cover for MRSA is increasingly being given, e.g. vancomycin 1g iv over 1h or teicoplanin 400mg IV. It is mandatory
  if the patient is known to be colonized.

Treatment of infection

Surgical site infection

- This is identified by:
  - skin redness;
  - pain;
  - swelling;
  - fever;
  - purulent discharge.
- Inflammatory markers, leucocyte count, and C-reactive protein will be elevated and can be monitored to assess response to treatment.
- Specimens must be taken for microbiological culture: wound swab and blood culture, as well as from sputum, urine, and central catheters if appropriate.
- Broad-spectrum antibiotics are given until culture and sensitivity results are available, when the antibiotic should be changed to narrow-spectrum, e.g. changing from cefuroxime to flucloxacillin if a flucloxacillin-sensitive S. aureus is grown from the wound swab. If MRSA is likely it is sensible to start with a glycopeptide. The duration depends on the response to treatment and if an organism is identified. A stop or review date should be stated at the outset. Changing from IV to PO treatment is often appropriate after 48h but depends on the response. The dose of antibiotic may need adjustment in patients with renal failure.
- Antibiotics only form one part of the treatment of surgical site infection. A collection requires effective drainage; wet necrotic tissue should be debrided and infected lines removed. Advice from the microbiologist and protocols are important because the epidemiology of infection and resistance varies from place to place.

Extremity ulceration

Ulcers support mixed bacterial communities that can include large numbers of staphylococci, streptococci, pseudomonads, coliforms, and anaerobes. These organisms will not be cleared by antibiotics as resistant strains will emerge.

The underlying cause needs to be diagnosed and treated. If skin grafting is planned beta-haemolytic streptococci and pseudomonads should be eliminated by topical antimicrobial agents, e.g. povidone–iodine or silver sulfadiazine. If there is gross contamination with large amounts of slough, preliminary surgical debridement will be required.

Extremity necrosis

The aim is to keep the necrosis dry or render it dry so that it mummifies and ultimately autoamputates.

- Exposure rather than bandaging.
- Maintain non-weight-bearing.
- Regular spraying with povidone–iodine dry powder.
- Bathing in potassium permanganate solution.

Some sogginess at the transition zone can be accepted but if there is cellulitis of the adjacent viable skin then antibiotics are indicated. Otherwise antibiotics are best avoided to prevent emergence of resistant strains.

Osteomyelitis

Diagnosis

- Suspect if an ulcer probes to bone.
- Common in diabetic foot infection.
- Swollen red sausage-like appearance of a toe.
- X-ray changes (localized loss of bone density, cortical outline).
- MRI scan (T1 sequence ↓ signal, STIR sequence ↑ uptake).
- Positive cultures from debrided bone or adjacent deep tissue.

Management

- Drain abscesses.
- Debride soft tissue necrosis.
- Remove dead bone or floating fragments.
- Send deep tissue and bone for culture.
- Antibiotics.

If there are no signs of an abscess or deep tissue necrosis a conservative approach may be tried. 3 months of antibiotics with good bone pentration, such as clindamycin, ciprofloxacin, rifampicin, and sodium fucidate, will be required. MRSA infections can be treated with appropriate IV antibiotics at home if there is a community IV service. The patient has a tunnelled central line or PICC line inserted prior to discharge from hospital.

An associated ulcer should be regularly debrided. If after 3 months the ulcer fails to heal and it still probes to bone then the underlying bone needs resection. This may require a toe amputation or metatarsal head resection.

Wet gangrene

Strict anaerobes such as *Clostridium*, *Bacteroides*, and *Peptostreptococci* produce a cocktail of destructive extracellular enzymes that allow invasion into deep tissues with extensive tissue necrosis. Gangrene has the potential for extensive migration. Rapid surgical control by amputation is therefore required to halt its spread.

Vascular surgery and prosthetics

The immune system cannot clear organisms from implanted prosthetic graft material. Once the foreign material is contaminated the infection can be impossible to clear without removing the graft. Infection with *Staphylococcus aureus* will present early with obvious wound infection and purulent discharge with systemic illness. MRSA is becoming the most prevalent cause of graft infection. Infection with *Staphylococcus epidermidis* seeded on to the graft at the time of implantation may not be apparent for up to 1 year. In such cases infections tend to present with non-specific symptoms and signs such as malaise, sweats, or fever before more obvious local signs become apparent:

• pseudoaneurysm;
• perigraft fluid collection;
• graft cutaneous fistula;
• aorto-enteric fistula;
• perigraft inflammation;
• graft thrombosis;
• bleeding from fistula to graft anastomosis.

Ideally, graft excision and extra-anatomic bypass are required to rid the patient of infection but removing a prosthetic graft often requires extensive surgery and it may prove difficult to provide an alternative conduit to maintain blood flow. The patient may die or lose a limb as a consequence. Attempts at conservative management have been tried with the aims of containing the infection and delaying the known complications of graft rupture and fistulation. Cure of infection is unlikely. Long-term systemic antibiotics can be effective if the organism concerned is of low virulence. In-situ replacement with antibiotic-soaked grafts or autologous vein after wide local debridement has been reported to be successful in selected cases.

Mycotic aneurysms

Definition A native artery aneurysm caused by infection.

Causes
- Endocarditis (haematological seeding).
- Traumatic innoculation (dirty needles, drug addicts, arterial lines).
- *Salmonella* (atherosclerotic vessels).
- Local spread (abscesses or osteomyelitis).

Clinical findings
- Fever.
- Warm and tender pulsatile mass (rapidly enlarging).
- Collapse (in the case of rupture).
- Saccular rather than fusiform shape on imaging.
- History of sepsis.
- Blood culture (only 50% positive).
  - *Staphylococcus*, 30%.
  - *Salmonellla*, 10%.
  - *Streptococcus*, 10%.

Recognition of the likely infective aetiology is essential in appropriate management. On the other hand, remember the possibility of a vascular connection in the pulsatile 'groin abscess'—get a duplex scan before 'incision and drainage'!

Treatment
- Depends on the site of the aneurysm.
- High dose antibiotics.
- Control and excision of the aneurysm if possible.
- Send wall of artery for culture.
- Revascularization only if necessary.
  - A non-essential artery, e.g. radial, can be tied off.
  - Femoral reconstruction in drug addicts is not advised. Collaterals will develop around a ligated common femoral, superficial femoral, or profunda artery in younger patients.
- Avoid prosthetics unless extra-anatomic route.
- If prosthetic unavoidable:
  - bond with rifampicin;
  - prolonged systemic antibiotics.

Complications of antibiotic treatment

Antibiotics alter the normal flora of the host and may lead to a number of problems.

Clostridium difficile **diarrhoea**

- This is usually acquired in hospital in patients who have received antibiotics.
- About 3% of healthy adults carry the organism in the large bowel.
- Hospital environments become contaminated with spores of this organism. The spores can survive for a long time and require enhanced environmental cleaning with chlorine disinfectant to be killed.
- Susceptible patients become infected by hand to mouth contamination either from the environment, health care workers, or cross-infection from affected patients. Alcohol hand gel does not kill the spores.
- In a host who has reduced intestinal flora, *C. difficile* multiplies and produces two toxins (A and B) that damage the enterocytes and cause diarrhoea. Severe cases develop colitis and a pseudomembrane.
- Affected patients should be isolated. Treatment is to stop the broad-spectrum antibiotic and give oral metronidazole or second-line vancomycin. Acidophilus lactobacillus tablets can be given to restore the intestinal bacterial flora. Patients can be advised to take live yoghurt when given antibiotics to reduce the risk of this condition.

Fungal infections

Patients with tunnelled lines or indwelling catheters are particularly susceptible to candidal infection. Patients may become systemically unwell if there is candidal septicaemia. Active treatment with antifungals will be required, e.g. fluconazole.

Resistant organisms

The continuing emergence of resistant strains of micro-organisms is a threat to the welfare of current and future patients. It is believed that the inappropriate use and overprescribing of antibiotics are in part responsible. It is therefore important to follow the principles for managing infections as outlined above, to adhere to local antibiotic policies, and to seek microbiological advice where appropriate.

Graft material in bypass grafting

Types of graft material

Four types of graft material are available: autograft; allograft; xenograft; and prosthetic material. Choice of which to use will depend on availability, particularly of autografts, and the clinical situation.

Autografts

- Autografts are portions of the patient's own vessels harvested from one site to be used as a conduit elsewhere. This is usually superficial vein, but deep vein or artery may be used.
- The suitability of autologous vein should be assessed preoperatively by duplex ultrasound, to ensure adequate length and a minimum diameter of 4mm throughout the segment to be used as well as the absence of deep venous dysfunction in that limb.
- It is useful to mark the course of the vein at the same time to facilitate harvesting.
- If no single segment of vein of adequate length and diameter is available, composite vein may be constructed by end-to-end anastomosis of multiple segments.
- Occasionally, large calibre vein grafts are required, such as in aortic repair when it is wished to avoid prosthetic material. Under these circumstances, superficial vein may be split longitudinally and sutured in a spiral form, producing a shorter tube of greater diameter. Alternatively, the superficial femoral vein can be used.

Greater saphenous vein (GSV)
- Most frequently used autologous vein graft.
- Usually of sufficient length and calibre for bypasses from groin to popliteal or crural vessels.
- May be used reversed or non-reversed after destruction of valves with a valvulotome. If non-reversed, may be left in situ (with tributaries ligated) or harvested and tunnelled deeply.
- Where ipsilateral GSV is unavailable, consideration should be given to use of vein from the contralateral limb for infrageniculate bypass.
- Palma bypass uses the GSV as a venous cross-over graft from one groin to the other for relief of venous obstruction secondary to ilio-femoral deep vein thrombosis.

Lesser saphenous vein (LSV)
- May be used as an alternative to GSV where this is unsuitable or has been harvested previously.
- Can be harvested with the patient prone or supine.
- Used preferentially for short grafts in the popliteal region, such as repair of popliteal aneurysms or intimal tears. When a posterior approach to the popliteal vessels is employed, harvest of the LSV is particularly convenient.

Arm vein
- May be used where there is no suitable leg vein available but there is a strong indication for the use of vein rather than prosthetic material.
- Cephalic and basilic veins are most often used.

- If forearm veins unsuitable, cephalic and basilic veins can be harvested in continuity with the antecubital vein and the valves lysed on one side of this loop (see Fig. 11.1).

Deep vein Use of the superficial femoral or popliteal veins as a conduit in the absence of suitable superficial vein has been described, with comparable patency to superficial vein and no long-term disability to the limb. It has been suggested (although not widely adopted) that deep vein should be used as the primary conduit for femoro-popliteal bypass grafts, retaining the greater saphenous vein for future distal bypass.

Artery Arterial autografts are rarely employed. However, use of radial artery autografts for reconstruction of the internal carotid artery has been described.

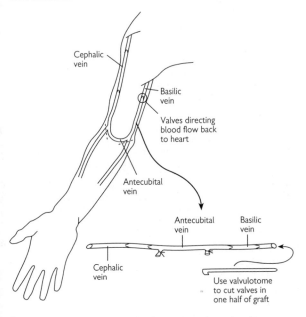

Fig 11.1 Harvesting of cephalic and basilic veins in continuous loop for extra length.

Allografts

Allografts are tissues taken from another individual of the same species.

Arterial allografts

- Preserved by irradiation or freeze-drying.
- Risks include:
  - occlusion;
  - aneurysm formation and rupture;
  - transmission of viruses and prion diseases;
  - rejection.
- Rarely used.

Venous allografts

- Preserved using DSMO or frozen with liquid nitrogen.
- Many of the same potential problems as arterial grafts including the risk of infection, aneurysmal dilatation, and rejection.
- Results are generally poor.

Human umbilical vein

- Preserved by glutaraldehyde-tanning.
- Particularly prone to aneurysmal dilatation.
- Patency inferior to that of saphenous vein grafts in femoro-above-knee popliteal bypass but equivalent to ePTFE.

Xenografts

- Xenografts are tissues derived from other species.
- The use of decellularized bovine carotid artery and, more recently, bovine ureter for peripheral arterial bypass has been described. Some units have described 1-year graft patency rates for grafts to the popliteal artery using bovine carotid artery that are comparable to those of ePTFE grafts.
- Such xenografts may in the future be used as frameworks to be populated by human endothelial cells to form bioprosthetic grafts.
- Concern remains regarding the risk of transmission of viral or prion diseases from other species into humans.

Prosthetic grafts

The commonest prosthetic materials employed in vascular grafts are expanded polytetrafluoroethylene (ePTFE) and polyurethane (Dacron).

ePTFE

- Available in a variety of lengths and diameters (from 4mm diameter upwards), as well as custom configurations such as axillo-bifemoral grafts. Its inner surface is smoother and less thrombogenic than Dacron. Some grafts have carbon lining the lumen to reduce thrombogenicity further.
- Can be obtained with external reinforcing rings to prevent kinking and occlusion of grafts that cross joints. These may be separate from the graft (allowing some rings to be stripped away) or integral.
- Suitable for infrainguinal bypass (including both above- and below-knee femoro-popliteal bypass) and extra-anatomic bypass such as femoro-femoral cross-over, axillo-femoral, and axillo-axillary bypass.

- For infrageniculate bypass, the distal anastomosis should incorporate some form of vein cuff.
- ePTFE grafts are available with pre-shaped hoods for the distal anastomosis in infrageniculate bypass as an alternative to fashioning of a vein cuff.

Polyurethane (Dacron) grafts

- Available in woven or knitted forms. The fibres of the woven material are much closer together with reduced porosity compared to the knitted form. However, the resultant graft is stiffer. The knitted graft is more flexible, but in the past its looser construction meant that these grafts had to be pre-clotted prior to use to prevent excessive blood leakage through the graft when first implanted. This problem has now been addressed by impregnation of the graft with collagen, albumin, or gelatin during manufacture.
- Most suitable for aorto-iliac reconstruction, though may also be used for extra-anatomic bypasses such as femoro-femoral bypass or axillo-femoral bypass.
- Grafts are available impregnated with silver, or antibiotics such as rifampicin, to be used when there is high risk of graft infection. However, there is little data to support the efficacy of such measures.

Graft patency rates

- Prosthetic grafts have excellent patency rates in aorto-iliac reconstructions, where the blood flow rates are high and conduits are of large diameter. Aorto-iliac bypass for occlusive disease has 5-year primary patency rates of greater than 80%.
- For infrainguinal bypass, the use of autologous vein grafts remains the gold standard. Five-year patency for femoro-popliteal bypass grafts (both above and below knee) using autologous GSV is around 70%, compared to around 40% for ePTFE grafts, although early patency rates are similar.
- For infrapopliteal bypass, the superiority of vein versus prosthetic graft is even more apparent, with 4-year primary patency rates of 50% for vein versus 10–20% for ePTFE. Where there is obligate use of a prosthetic graft to the infrapopliteal vessels, this should be in combination with a vein cuff (e.g. Miller cuff or St. Mary's boot) or patch (e.g. Taylor patch) at the distal anastomosis,
- There is no evidence that the use of reversed autologous vein rather than an in situ technique has any effect on graft patency. However, the use of non-reversed vein (either in situ or tunnelled) for infrapopliteal bypass may give a better size match between graft and native vessel at each anastomosis, making the procedure technically easier.
- Cephalic vein bypasses have similar patency rates to GSV for femoro-popliteal bypass (5-year patency of ~70%).
- Cryopreserved vein allografts perform poorly with 1-year patency of < 30%.

Graft infection

- Graft infection probably occurs in 0.5–2% of reconstructions. Venous grafts are seldom affected—another reason for the preferential use of autologous vein when available. The vast majority of graft infections are seen in prosthetic grafts.
- Silver-impregnated and rifampicin-bonded grafts are purported to have increased resistance to graft infection, but there is little evidence to support this assertion.
- Prosthetic grafts should not be implanted in an infected field. Where an infected prosthetic graft has to be removed, this should ideally be replaced with an autologous vein graft. If suitable vein is not available, prosthetic material may be used in an extra-anatomic bypass that avoids the infected area.
- In the aorto-iliac segment, where it is unlikely that autologous vein of sufficient calibre will be available, the graft may be replaced with a silver or antibiotic-impregnated graft. Alternatively, extra-anatomic bypass with a prosthetic axillo-bifemoral graft may be carried out.
- Arterial allografts have been used in the setting of graft infection. They are not completely resistant to infection themselves, however and are prone to dilatation and aneurysm formation.

Graft surveillance

- When the intima of a vein graft is subjected to arterial pressure, intimal hyperplasia may result. Areas of intimal hyperplasia may give rise to graft stensoses and subsequent graft occlusion. There is clear evidence that duplex ultrasound graft surveillance can improve secondary graft patency by detecting haemodynamically significant graft stenoses. These can then be treated before they result in graft occlusion.
- Prosthetic grafts do not possess an intima and consequently are not affected by intimal hyperplasia. Graft occlusion is likely to be as a result of progression of in-flow or run-off disease. There is no evidence that surveillance of prosthetic grafts is of benefit.

Techniques of vascular surgery

Exposure of the aorta

Transperitoneal approach

Commonest approach. Allows inspection of peritoneal contents.

Patient position Supine.

Incision

There are two alternative incisions.

1 Vertical midline from xiphisternum to just above symphisis pubis
- Quick, good access to proximal aorta up to SMA and down to iliac arteries.
- Aorta can be controlled at diaphragm if necessary (mobilize left lobe of liver and divide right crus of diaphragm) but access between here and SMA difficult because of pancreas unless spleen and pancreas mobilized completely over to the right.

2 Transverse just above/below umbilicus
- Less respiratory compromise postoperatively.
- In tall thin patient access to upper aorta and distal iliac vessels may be more difficult.

Steps
1 Full laparotomy in elective case.
2 Move small bowel to right of abdomen to expose duodenal–jejunal flexure.
3 Incise retroperitoneum around 4th part of duodenum to mobilize it off aorta.
4 Clear tissue from anterior wall of aorta at this level and then dissect up in same plane until you reach left renal vein crossing aorta (don't mistake inferior mesenteric vein for the renal vein—the former runs much more superficially and obliquely; the latter is closely applied to the aorta (Fig. 12.1)). This gives you a guide to the position of the renal arteries so that an infrarenal clamp can be applied. *Note*: occasionally the left renal veins runs behind the aorta in which case the level of dissection has to be decided from the renal arteries found on clearing either side of the aorta.
5 Clear the sides of the aorta just below the renal arteries until you can feel the vertebra behind on both sides.
6 Incise the posterior peritoneum vertically down the front of the aorta and into the pelvis from the aortic bifurcation.
7 Lift up the leaves of peritoneum on either side to access the iliac arteries, watching out for iliac veins behind the arteries as you mobilize the vessels.

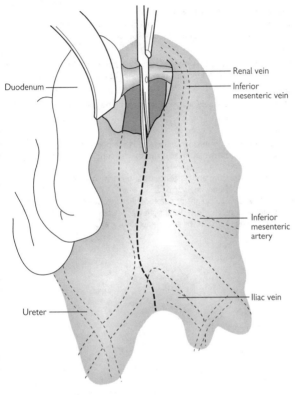

Fig. 12.1 Exposure of the aorta via a transperitoneal approach.

Retroperitoneal approach

May be useful when there are peritoneal adhesions, a colostomy, inflammatory aneurysm, or respiratory compromise.

Patient position

Upper body turned to right with sandbag under left flank and left arm supported above body on arm support (Fig. 12.2).

Incision

Tip of 9th rib obliquely across abdomen below umbilicus to right iliac fossa.

Steps

1　Deepen incision through muscle to reach peritoneum.
2　Open plane between muscle and peritoneum in post-inferior wound edge.
3　Push peritoneum and its contents anteriorly to reach aorta, usually leaving left kidney undisturbed.
4　Gives access to origins of common iliac arteries for control but difficult to reach more distal right iliac vessels for aorto-iliac graft. Tunnelling to groins for aorto-bifemoral grafts is feasible.

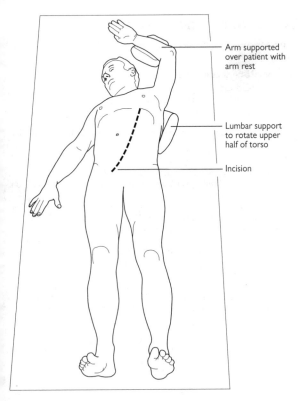

Fig. 12.2 Position of patient for a retroperitoneal approach to the aorta.

Exposure of iliac arteries

Transperitoneal approach See transperitoneal approach in 'Exposure of the aorta', p. 192.

Extraperitoneal approach

Useful to avoid major insult of transperitoneal approach when grafting from here distally or performing an iliac endarterectomy.

Patient position Supine.

Incision Curved following skin crease in iliac fossa 4–5cm above inguinal ligament.

Steps

1   Deepen incision, splitting external oblique between fibres and dividing internal oblique and transversus in line with the skin incision to expose peritoneum.

2   Develop plane between peritoneum and muscle to allow peritoneum and its contents to be mobilized superomedially to allow access to the retroperitoneum.

3   Feel for the hard cord of the iliac arteries, tracing the external iliac artery from the inguinal ligament in order to identify it.

4   Expose the iliac arteries as far as the aortic bifurcation if necessary. The internal iliac can be found as a deep branch taking off posteromedially from the common iliac artery. Watch out for the iliac veins posterior to the arteries when slinging the vessel. Look out for the ureter crossing the common iliac bifurcation (see Fig. 12.3).

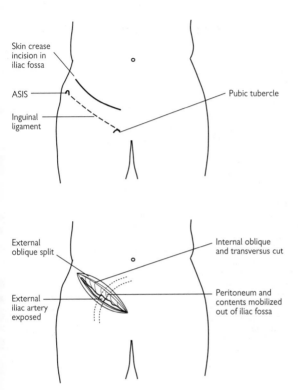

Fig. 12.3 Extraperitoneal exposure of iliac arteries.

Exposure of common femoral artery

Patient position Supine.

Incision

Either
- Vertical over the CFA from approximately 1cm above level of inguinal ligament to 5cm below. If no femoral pulse palpable, position is 2/3 down line from anterior superior iliac spine to pubic tubercle. Quick simple approach, but crosses groin almost at 90° leading to patient discomfort and tendency to dehisce.

Or
- Oblique incision following skin creases over middle third of inguinal ligament then curving down into thigh along line of GSV. Probably causes less discomfort and better healing (see Fig. 12.4).

Steps

1 Deepen incision through Scarpa's fascia.

2a In vertical approach, continue deepening with sharp dissection through deep fascia until anterior surface of femoral artery is reached making sure that incision stays over the artery as far as possible. Small crossing veins may be encountered but usually nothing else of significance.

2b In the oblique approach, reflect Scarpa's fascia so that you can make a vertical incision in the deep fascia over the CFA (and so avoid cutting across the lymphatics coursing up medial to the CFA) and continue as above.

3 Once the anterior surface of the artery is exposed at one point, clear proximally up to inguinal ligament and distally for length of incision placing self-retaining retractor with blades on deep fascia to improve exposure.

4 Clear sides of artery just below inguinal ligament and pass silastic sling around at this level.

5 Look for narrowing of artery where it changes from common femoral to superficial femoral artery (see Fig. 12.5). Clear either side of proximal part of SFA and pass silastic sling around at this point.

6 Lift up the two slings to expose the relatively posterior-lateral origin of the profunda artery (there may be more than one) as you dissect along the medial and lateral surfaces of the CFA. Pass sling around profunda origin (if access is diffiicult pass the sling across the back of the CFA below the level of the profunda and then bring it back above the origin).

7 Double sling any other arterial branches in the field with 0 silk or other braided tie.

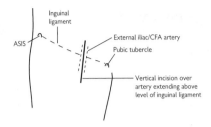

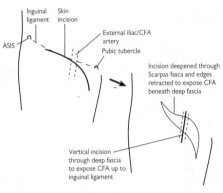

Fig. 12.4 Alternative incisions for CFA exposure. (a) Vertical incision; (b) oblique incision.

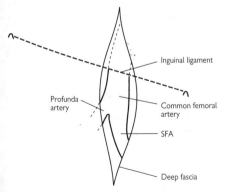

Fig. 12.5 Exposure of the CFA, SFA, and the profunda artery.

Exposure of popliteal artery

Medial approach to above-knee section

Used when a supine position is needed, e.g. for bypass from the groin or for harvesting of GSV.

Patient position

Supine with leg externally rotated at hip and flexed at knee, supported on a sandbag. Surgeon on opposite side of table facing medial aspect of leg.

Incision

Feel for posterior medial edge of femur and use this to place the incision along the distal 12cm of femur curving posteriorly 1–2cm along proximal part of femoral condyle, avoiding damage to the GSV.

Steps

1 Incise deep fascia parallel with anterior border of sartorius.
2 Dissect in the plane that opens up easily between the anterior border of sartorius and the femur. Feel with your finger for the firm cord of the popliteal artery posterior to the femur, watching out for the major branches of the sciatic nerve.
3 Use a deep-bladed self-retaining retractor to maintain exposure of the vascular bundle, which contains both popliteal artery and vein with several crossing arterial branches/venous tributaries that often have to be divided to allow separation of the popliteal vessels and slinging of the artery (see Fig. 12.6).

Medial approach to below-knee section

Used when a supine position is needed, e.g. for bypass from the groin or for harvesting of GSV, and the proximal popliteal artery is diseased.

Patient position

Supine with leg externally rotated at hip and flexed at knee. Surgeon on opposite side of table facing medial aspect of leg.

Incision

1cm posterior to and parallel with posterior medial edge of tibia starting approximately 6cm distal to knee joint, approximately 12cm long. Avoid damage to the GSV.

Steps

1 Deepen incision through deep fascia and between gastrocnemius and back of tibia (see Fig. 12.7).
2 Feel for vascular bundle on back of tibia and dissect down to this, watching out for tibial nerve.
3 Often two popliteal veins run alongside the artery with a number of arterial branches and venous tributaries crossing that have to be divided so that the artery can be separated and slung.

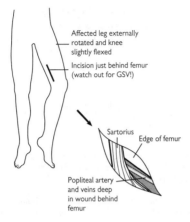

Affected leg externally rotated and knee slightly flexed

Incision just behind femur (watch out for GSV!)

Sartorius

Edge of femur

Popliteal artery and veins deep in wound behind femur

Fig. 12.6 Medial exposure of above-knee popliteal artery.

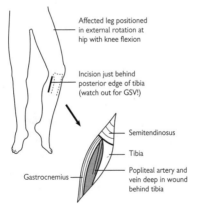

Affected leg positioned in external rotation at hip with knee flexion

Incision just behind posterior edge of tibia (watch out for GSV!)

Semitendinosus

Tibia

Gastrocnemius

Popliteal artery and vein deep in wound behind tibia

Fig. 12.7 Medial exposure of below-knee popliteal artery.

Posterior approach to popliteal artery

Used for access to above- and/or below-knee popliteal artery when access to anterior aspect of limb and GSV not required, e.g. for popliteal aneurysm or localized trauma to the popliteal artery. The LSV can be used for local bypass surgery.

Patient position Prone.

Incision

Sigmoid with approximately 6cm long vertical components posterior-medial proximally and posterior-lateral distally, joined by horizontal part across posterior knee crease.

Steps

1   Deepen incision through deep fascia to reach the popliteal fossa.
2   Feel for neurovascular bundle. The sciatic nerve and its branches will be most superficial followed by the popliteal vein, then artery (see Fig. 12.5).
3   Mobilize nerve and vein laterally to expose and sling the artery at the level required with division of venous tributaries as required.

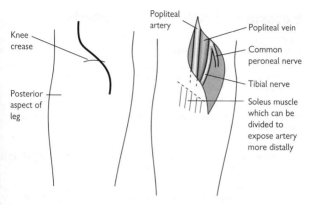

Fig. 12.8 Posterior approach to popliteal artery.

Exposure of calf and foot arteries

Medial approach to tibio-peroneal artery and origins of the three crural arteries

This approach gives reasonable exposure of the proximal third of the posterior tibial and peroneal arteries but access to only the first 1–2cm of the anterior tibial artery.

Patient position

Supine with hip externally rotated and knee flexed and resting on a sandbag or similar support.

Incision

In the upper medial calf parallel and 1cm posterior to posterior border of upper third of tibia, approximately 12–15cm long.

Steps

1   Incise deep fascia along length of wound and open up plane between gastrocnemius and back of tibia.
2   Feel for popliteal artery behind tibia and dissect this out, being careful to avoid tibial nerve and to preserve popliteal vein (although several tributaries will need to be divided to allow access to the artery).
3   Follow the popliteal artery distally as it gives off the anterior tibial artery anteriorly, continues as the tibio-peroneal artery, then gives off the posterior tibial artery posteriorly and continues as the peroneal artery. If necessary take soleus muscle off the back of the tibia to expose the arteries distally. At least one anterior tibial vein often has to be sacrificed to reach the origin of the anterior tibial artery (see Fig. 12.9).

Anterior tibial artery

This can be exposed at its origin via a medial approach (see above) and anywhere along its subsequent course in the anterior compartment (Fig. 12.10).

Patient position Supine.

Incision

Vertical over centre of anterior compartment, approximately 5cm long.

Steps

1   Feel for indentation between the two muscles (tibialis anterior and extensorum digitorum longus) as you move the hallux and then the ankle in extension and flexion and incise deep fascia along this line.
2   Separate the two muscles to find the anterior tibial artery and veins lying at their base.
3   Several tributaries of the two veins may need dividing to free the artery.

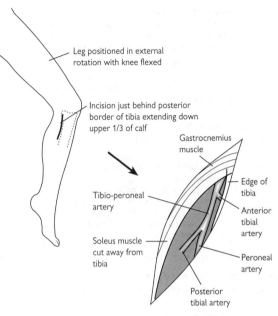

Fig. 12.9 Exposure of the tibio-peroneal stem and origins of the crural arteries.

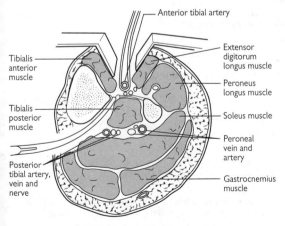

Fig. 12.10 Exposure of the anterior tibial artery.

Peroneal artery in distal calf

Sometimes the peroneal artery is the only conserved artery in the lower leg and, although it does not run directly into the foot, it sends a significant contribution to both the posterior and anterior tibial distal circulations and proves useful as the recipient artery for a distal bypass graft.

Patient position

Supine with the leg internally rotated if possible (slight knee flexion on a sandbag or similar support may help).

Incision

Vertical along palpable edge of fibula, approximately 10cm long with distal end about 6cm proximal to tip of lateral malleolus.

Steps

1 Incise on to fibula for the full length of the skin incision, anterior to peroneus longus and brevis.
2 Use a periosteal elevator to lift periosteum from full circumference of fibula for about 6cm in the centre of the wound.
3 Use bone cutters or Gigli saw to divide fibula at each end of exposed portion so that 5–6cm length of bone can be removed.
4 Gently make a longitudinal incision in the periosteum on the far side of the fibula exposed by this action to find the peroneal artery and its attendant veins just underneath (see Fig. 12.11).

Posterior tibial artery at the ankle

The artery can be followed into the foot from this incision.

Patient position

Supine with leg externally rotated.

Incision

Vertical approximately 1cm behind medial malleolus and extending approximately 5cm up behind distal tibia.

Steps

1 Incise deep fascia in line of skin incision.
2 The posterior tibial artery lies between flexor digitorum longus anteriorly and the posterior tibial nerve behind, just under the deep fascia.
3 Its venae comitantes may need to be divided to isolate the artery.

Dorsalis pedis artery

Patient position Supine.

Incision

Vertical or sigmoid incision extending from just distal to the midpoint anteriorly between the two malleoli for about 4cm.

Step

• Dissect down between the tendons of extensor hallucis longus and extensor digitorum longus to find the artery with its two veins.

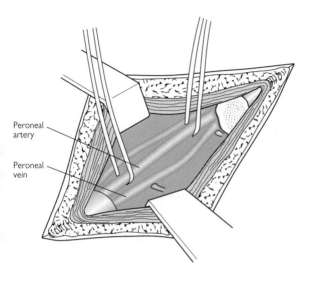

Peroneal
artery

Peroneal
vein

Fig. 12.11 Exposure of the distal peroneal artery.

Exposure of carotid artery

Patient position Supine with operating table 'broken' so that the upper torso is elevated. The neck needs to be extended; the head rotated to other side and on a head ring.

Incision
Either
- Obliquely down anterior border of sternomastoid.

Or
- Transversely in the line of the skin creases, centred over the anterior border of sternomastoid at the level of the carotid bifurcation (either marked preoperatively or approximately 2cm below mandible).

Steps
1   Use sharp dissection to deepen the incision through platysma.
2   In the transverse incision elevate platysma flaps either side of the incision up to the mandible and to about 4cm below the incision line.
3   In both incisions then incise along the anterior border of sternomastoid to expose the internal jugular vein.
4   Approach the carotid vessels either anterior or posterior to the jugular vein (an anterior approach will require division of more venous tributaries including the facial vein).
5   Divide the thick carotid sheath over the common carotid artery in the proximal part of the wound, looking out for the vagus nerve, which usually lies behind the artery but occasionally runs across its anterior surface.
6   Extend the incision in the carotid sheath up to the carotid bifurcation and up the external carotid artery, identified by its branches, in particular the first—the superior thyroid, which takes off anterior-medially.
7   Clear the proximal common carotid and place a silastic sling around it.
8   Clear the proximal external carotid artery just distal to the superior thyroid artery and place a silastic sling around it. Watch out for the hypoglossal nerve which runs across both internal and external carotid arteries. Double sling the superior thyroid artery with a 0 silk or similar braided tie.
9   Find the distal internal carotid artery, usually posterior and sometimes deep to the external carotid artery, again looking out for the hypoglossal nerve. In a retrojugular approach watch out for the accessory nerve high in the wound. Try and reach the portion of internal carotid artery beyond the diseased segment where the hard plaque in the wall gives way to a soft often tortuous vessel. Clear the artery gently at this point and place a silastic sling around it but ensure that the clip on the sling cannot slip and inadvertently cause arterial occlusion (you may wish to secure just one end with a clip on to the drapes and leave the other end free).

10 Very gently completely mobilize the bifurcation region between these slings. Rough handling of this region may lead to cerebral embolization from a diseased carotid bulb. Watch out for bradycardia and hypotension because of carotid sinus nerve stimulation—this can be blocked with injection into the tissue between the bifurcation with 1mL 1% lidocaine. The ansa cervicalis lies on front of the carotid vessels and may need to be divided for access (it is much smaller than the vagus and has a contribution from the hypoglossal nerve (see Fig. 12.12).

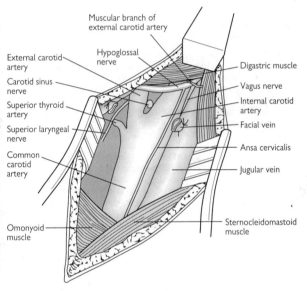

Fig. 12.12 Exposure of the carotid bifurcation.

Exposure of subclavian artery

Supraclavicular approach

Patient position

Supine with neck extended and head turned to opposite side on a head ring. Useful to have ipsilateral upper arm also prepped and forearm/hand wrapped in stockingette and placed on draped chest so that it can be moved to open up the supraclavicular fossa if necessary either by rotation or by depressing the shoulder.

Incision

1cm above middle third of clavicle.

Steps

1   Cut through platysma and, deep to this, cut through clavicular head of sternomastoid to expose scalenus anterior lying deep to it.

2   Mobilize the scalene fat pad and the underlying phrenic nerve off the anterior surface of scalenus anterior before dividing this muscle.

3   Look out for the subclavian artery running transversely deep to scalenus anterior (take care if using diathermy to divide the muscle).

4   Mobilize the artery gently and sling. It is often necessary to control the internal mammary artery (running inferiorly), the thyrocervical trunk (running superiorly), and the costocervical trunk running anteriorly from this part of the subclavian artery. Look out for cords of the brachial plexus that surround the artery laterally and for the thoracic duct, which crosses the proximal part of the left subclavian artery on its way to join the subclavian vein. Medial retraction (± extension of incision) will expose common carotid artery and vertebral artery (see Fig. 12.13).

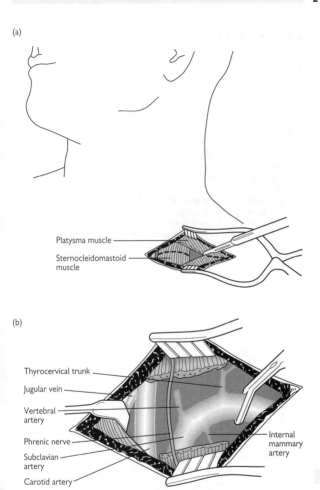

(a)

Platysma muscle

Sternocleidomastoid muscle

(b)

Thyrocervical trunk

Jugular vein

Vertebral artery

Phrenic nerve

Subclavian artery

Carotid artery

Internal mammary artery

Fig. 12.13 Supraclavicular exposure of the subclavian artery. (a) Site of incision; (b) deep exposure.

Exposure of axillary artery

Patient position
Supine with arm extended out to the side at 90° on an arm board.

Incision
A horizontal incision is made below and parallel to the middle third of the clavicle.

Steps
1 Deepen the incision through the subcutaneous fascia and that covering the pectoralis major muscle.
2 Separate the fibres of pectoralis major by blunt dissection.
3 Divide the deep fascia to expose the pectoralis minor muscle. Divide this using diathermy in its tendinous portion, close to its insertion into the coracoid process. Division of this muscle exposes the second part of the axillary artery, which can now be dissected free and controlled with vascular slings, along with any branches seen. The axillary vein, anterior and inferior to the artery, may be adherent to the artery or may not be seen at all (see Fig. 12.14).

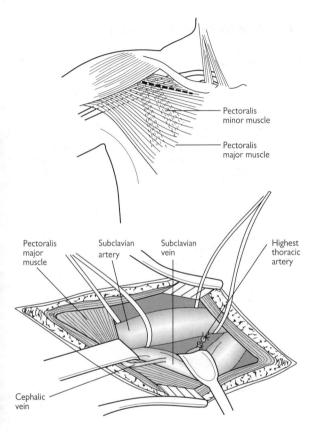

Fig. 12.14 Exposure of the axillary artery.

Exposure of brachial artery

Patient position

Supine with arm supported out on a large arm board or operating table.

Incision

Sigmoid over medial part of antecubital fossa (see Fig. 12.5).

Steps

1 Cut down on to and divide bicipital aponeurosis.
2 Find brachial artery just below.
3 Look out for median nerve, which crosses the anterior surface
of the artery to lie on its medial side possibly high in the wound
(see Fig. 12.15).

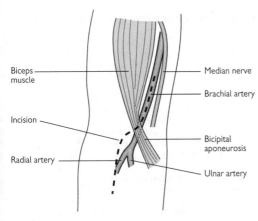

Fig 12.15 Exposure of the brachial artery.

Techniques for vascular anastomoses

Anastomotic sites

- These are usually decided in principle preoperatively on the basis of arterial imaging and severity of symptoms (rest pain/ischaemic tissue loss generally requires more extensive bypass grafting than claudication).
- There should be no obvious stenosis > 50% above the proximal anastomosis (this may not be haemodynamically significant but is likely to progress and will limit graft durability).
- Ideally there should be at least one vessel in continuity down to the ankle from the distal anastomosis but an extensive collateral run-off may be sufficient if it is the only option. Dependent duplex scanning will sometimes show a patent major vessel distally where angiography has shown no obvious site for a distal anastomosis.
- If the proposed site of the distal anastomosis in an infrainguinal bypass graft is uncertain from the preoperative angiogram or dependent duplex, an on-table angiogram may be planned in advance to give clearer views of the run-off. At operation, before exposing any other sites, expose the below-knee popliteal artery (if open on imaging) and inject 10–15mL 50% Niopam® via a 21G butterfly needle under X-ray screening. If the popliteal artery is occluded then expose one of the distal arteries at a possible anastomosis site, i.e. an open artery with possible run-off unclear on preoperative imaging. Sometimes no good run-off is found in which case there is no point in proceeding with a bypass graft.

General principles of anastomosis

- Vein grafts need minimal and gentle handling to prevent endothelial damage (in particular), which might promote thrombosis.
  - During mobilization, lift up with a sling or apply forceps to ligated tributaries, adherent connective tissue, or adventitia.
  - Once mobilized from its bed, make sure vein is kept moist with/in saline.
  - During anastomosis, avoid use of forceps on the vein if possible; apply only to the edge of vein that will be within suture line or to the adventitia while positioning the hood.
- Avoid loose fragments or flaps of plaque within the artery.
  - Remove or tack down flaps exposed at arteriotomy.
  - Make sure that, as far as possible, the needle is always passed from inside to outside of the arterial wall to avoid lifting plaque.
- If proximal arteriotomy is below the aortic bifurcation (and above this level if aortic pulsation appears weak), check 'run-in' before starting anastomosis by releasing controlling clamp for a second or two, checking that the systemic systolic BP is > 100mmHg first (ask the anaesthetist to put it up if necessary). Flow should be pulsatile and 'audible'. If it is not, you need to improve run-in before proceeding with anastomosis (e.g. by proximal endarterectomy, on-table proximal angioplasty, moving to a higher anastomosis site, or performing a proximal bypass graft to provide run-in to this site).

- Check run-off at distal arteriotomy before deciding on final length of graft prior to anastomosis. Inspect lumen of artery just beyond arteriotomy and flush the vessel distal to this with a syringe of heparin saline on a vascular cannula with the clamp removed—there should be very little resistance to instilling 20mL saline. It may be necessary to perform an on-table angiogram via the cannula to check for distal obstruction. If outflow is restricted this can be dealt with by local endarterectomy (being careful not to leave a distal flap unsecured), possibly via an extended arteriotomy, or by moving to a more distal anastomotic site below any obstruction.
- Avoid tension and compression in/on the graft.
  - Do not be tempted to stretch an inadequate length of graft to make it reach—it will tear off at one end and the lumen will be flattened and restricted.
  - Make sure you check graft length with the knee extended if the graft crosses this joint.
  - Check for constricting bands or graft angulation once flow is established (latter is common when running a superficial graft to the popliteal artery) and free up any tissue restraining the graft.
- Wound closure over a vascular anastomosis needs to be done with care.
  - Good haemostasis is important and, if there is persistent low volume oozing despite your best attempts at haemostasis, including protamine to reverse any heparin, then consider leaving a vacuum drain in the wound overnight. This happens particularly in a re-explored groin where there has been a lot of sharp dissection.
  - An exposed graft will become infected and an exposed vein graft will dry out and disrupt so make sure the graft is securely covered by subcutaneous tissue and skin.
  - Avoid use of forceps on the distal skin of the leg—fragile, elderly skin damaged by ischaemia and under tension if there is postoperative swelling will infarct easily at the wound edges leading to wound breakdown. Don't compound the problem with further injury.

Controlling the arteries

- There are clamps designed for arteries of all sizes. Use the appropriate type for the size of artery, e.g. aortic curved clamp, cushioned Fogarty clamps for medium-sized arteries and small Bulldog clamps, Heifitz clips, or similar for the small arteries. Be careful not to damage the arterial wall by putting on the adjustable clamps too firmly (2–3 steps on the ratchet is usually sufficient). Try to avoid cracking plaque with the clamp—this is unavoidable if the plaque is circumferential but, if it is localized posteriorly, then placing the clamp with one jaw on the posterior wall and one on the anterior wall may prevent cracking.
- Double slinging the artery with silastic slings under tension achieves good control in soft small vessels and may be less traumatic than clamping.

- Lumen occluding devices that slip inside the artery may be useful if the artery is too hard to compress with a clamp. In the large- to medium-sized arteries a Fogarty balloon catheter blown up in the artery via a 3-way tap to secure inflation works in the same way.
- A tourniquet (at 120mmHg) placed above the anastomosis site before skin incision will control bleeding unless the arteries are heavily calcified. This is particularly useful when you know that it will be difficult to gain control of the arteries before breaching the arterial lumen, e.g. with a large false aneurysm below the groin.

Bypass graft anastomosis

This can be either 'end-to-end' or 'end-to-side' depending on the con-figuration of the artery and graft. End-to-side will allow backperfusion in the artery. End-to-side is preferred if there is a serious size mismatch between the graft and arterial diameters.

End-to-end anastomosis

See Fig. 12.16.
- Transect artery obliquely.
- Cut graft to match. A mismatch in lumen diameters will cause angulation of the anastomosis (which does not matter if relatively small).
- Use a double-ended Prolene suture (see 'Anastomotic sutures', p. 222, for size) to secure the 'heel' of the graft to the 'toe' of the artery taking one needle from inside to out on the graft wall and the other from inside to out on the artery wall; then tying the suture. Rubbershod the two ends. Repeat the procedure with a new suture between the 'toe' of the graft and the 'heel' of the artery.
- Take one of the needles and place a continuous suture between artery and graft until a point halfway along that side of the anastomosis, controlling position of the graft and artery by moving the two rubbershod clamps on the unused suture ends. Place a rubbershod on the end of this suture. Take one of the needles from the other side of the anastomosis and run this as a continuous suture until this half of the anastomosis is finished and tie it to the the previous suture. Rubbershod the two used sutures.
- Repeat the procedure on the other side of the graft.

In this way there are four points in the suture line fixed by knots, so preventing 'purse stringing' of the anastomosis, which would narrow it.

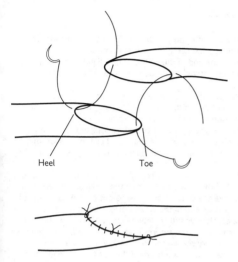

Fig 12.16 End-to-end anastomosis.

End-to-side anastomosis
See Fig. 12.17.
- Make a longitudinal arteriotomy in the middle of the exposed artery. Length should be approximately 1.5 × graft diameter.
- Create a 'hood' at the end of the graft that has slightly curving sides so that it is wider than a straight cut obliquely across the end of the graft would produce.
  - In a synthetic graft this is done by placing a curved clip obliquely across the end of the graft. Use a no. 11 blade cutting on to the concave side of the clamp to divide the graft.
  - In a vein graft it is usually easiest to make a longitudinal venotomy, using Potts scissors for a distance that matches the arteriotomy and then cut the corners in a curve round to the apex or 'toe' of the graft.
- Using a double-ended Prolene suture, pass both needles from outside to in on the heel of the graft either side of the midline. Rubbershod one suture and take the other from inside to out on the same side of the midline at the near end of the arteriotomy, leaving the suture slack. Proceed with a continuous suture between heel of graft and this side of the arteriotomy until three sutures have been placed, all left slack so that the graft and artery remain separated and you have a clear view for placing accurate sutures. Rubbershod the needle and repeat the process on the opposite side using the other needle. Pull this 'parachute' suture tight by alternately pulling on the two sutures and the graft, everting the suture edges (easier with vein than synthetic graft) (Fig 12.17).
- Rubbershod one of the sutures and continue the other suture line along the arteriotomy. As you approach the distal end adjust the stitch placement (to take up slack) or trim the graft if necessary to match graft to artery. Place 3–5 radiating sutures around the toe of the graft to secure it accurately to the far end of the arteriotomy so that the middle suture is in line with the arteriotomy. If necessary leave these five sutures slack to allow accurate suture placement; then draw the suture tight. Continue suturing until halfway along the other side; then rubbershod the suture. Take up the other needle and complete the anastomosis, tying the two suture ends together after reversing the direction of the last stitch so that the tie crosses the anastomotic line.

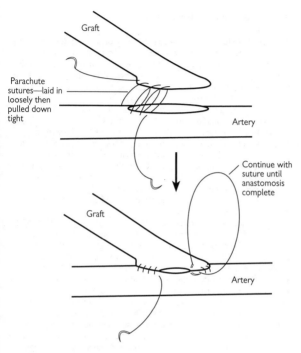

Fig. 12.17 End to side anastomosis.

Patch closure of an arteriotomy

See Fig. 12.18.

This usually follows a local endarterectomy or an embolectomy with a longitudinal arteriotomy and is used when direct closure of the artery would produce unacceptable narrowing. Synthetic material (e.g. PTFE or heparin-bonded Dacron) or locally harvested vein can be used. A vein patch takes longer to produce but is easier to suture, particularly in small or very thin-walled (post-endarterectomy) arteries. A vein patch is less likely to become infected (especially in an ulcerated leg). Vein should always be used, if possible, in small arteries, e.g. those below the popliteal, because it has less risk of thrombosis in these low flow sites.

- If using vein to patch, find a length of superficial vein at least 3mm in diameter to match the length of the arteriotomy. Ensure that any tributaries are ligated with 3/0 silk. Open the vein longitudinally and cut off the corners at each end so that there is a reasonably smooth convex curve of vein either side of the apex.
- If using synthetic material cut the same size and shape patch as described with vein.
- Using a double-ended Prolene or PTFE suture (if using a PTFE patch), take one of the needles through the apex at one end of the patch, passing from outside to in. Continue out through one end of the arteriotomy. Pull the suture so that you have equal ends and rubbershod one of them. Keep the patch and artery apart and using the needle on the other end , place two more loose sutures in a continuous suture line between the curved end of the patch and the end of the arteriotomy, placing radiating sutures around the latter. Place three sutures on the other side in a similar fashion, using the other needle and taking it first from outside to inside on the patch.
- Tighten this 'parachute' suture by pulling alternately on the two suture ends and on the graft, making sure that the patch and arterial edges are everted.
- Continue round the patch with a continuous suture, placing 3–5 radiating sutures around the other end of the arteriotomy. Stop halfway down the other side of the patch. Use the other needle to complete the suture line, tying the two ends together.

Anastomotic sutures

- Monofilament polypropylene sutures run through the tissues easily and allow several sutures to be left slack to allow a better view for accurate suturing before they are drawn up tight.
- PTFE suture is designed to plug the stitch holes (which tend to bleed) in PTFE by attaching the suture to a needle of the same size (rather than slightly bigger as in other sutures).
- Round-bodied needles are usually employed but may not penetrate calcified plaque in which case a specially designed cutting needle may be used.
- Suture size depends on thickness of the vessel walls. A rough guide would be:
  - 2/0 or 3/0 for aortic anastomoses;
  - 3/0 or 4/0 for iliac anastomosis;

- 4/0 or 5/0 (depending whether synthetic or vein graft) in the groin;
- 5/0 or 6/0 below the groin, depending on the graft material.

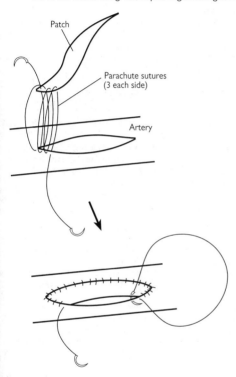

Fig. 12.18 Patch closure of an arteriotomy.

Techniques for haemostasis

Anastomotic bleeding

Poor suturing technique (widely spaced or loose sutures) will of course lead to bleeding. Sometimes, however, such problems arise even when the greatest of care is taken because of friable arteries that tear, calcified plaque that prevents you placing the suture where you would like it, and difficult access. The following techniques may help.

- When testing the anastomosis decide whether the blood comes from:
  - around most of the suture line (loose suture likely);
  - 1 or 2 specific points on the suture line where the stitches are too far apart;
  - an arterial tear related to a stitch hole.
- Reclamp before attempting repair.
- A loose suture will have to be dealt with either by pulling up the suture at one point to tighten the whole suture line and using a new stitch through the loop and the suture line to hold it tight (Fig. 12.19), or by resuturing over the previous suture line.
- If the suture line is bleeding at a single point use a 2/0 or 3/0 'z' stitch across the suture line to close the gap.
- If a stitch hole is bleeding:
  - use 3/0 Prolene as a 'z' stitch across the line of the tear, which is usually vertical (Fig. 12.20).
  - If a stitch hole continues to bleed consider repeating the 'z' stitch but taking the suture through a PTFE pledgelet or small piece of vein on its way to and from the arterial wall; the pledgelet/vein is pulled down on to the defect as the suture is tied securely over the top of it.
- In an aortic inlay anastomosis the posterior part of the suture line is sometimes difficult to inspect, although it is usually possible to roll the graft over to some extent for at least a limited view. Sometimes there is sufficient access to run a buttressing suture between graft and aortic

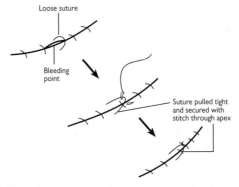

Loose suture

Bleeding point

Suture pulled tight and secured with stitch through apex

Fig. 12.19 Tightening a loose suture line.

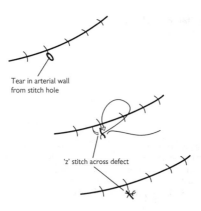

Fig. 12.20 Repair of an arterial tear from stitch hole.

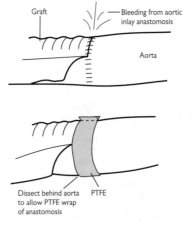

Fig. 12.21 Using PTFE 'wrap' to stop bleeding from aortic inlay anastomosis.

wall across the back. If you have inadequate access to do this, try
mobilizing the back wall of the aorta forward (dividing lumbar arteries
if necessary and taking care not to divide deeply penetrating
anastomotic sutures) and wrapping a length of PTFE (approximately
0.5–1cm wide) around it at the level of the anastomosis, securing it
anteriorly with 2/0 Prolene (Fig. 12.21). Occasionally it proves
impossible to identify the site of a significant bleeding point posteriorly
and the anastomosis has to be taken down and redone with a closer
suturing technique.

Managing iliac vein bleeding
- Iliac vein bleeding presents during surgery with profuse welling up of dark blood in the pelvis.
- Do not try and clamp blindly—you are likely to cause more damage.
- Apply pressure with a pack while you:
  - alert the anaesthetist;
  - round up good assistance
  - arrange satisfactory lighting and retraction;
  - get at least two suckers.
- Cautiously remove the pack while retracting the iliac artery if you have it slung and using suction. If bleeding is too profuse to see the bleeding point, reapply pressure with a pack and arm yourself with two swabs on spongeholders, applying these one at a time to where you imagine the iliac vein to lie above and below the bleeding points, compressing through the iliac artery if necessary. Move cautiously and reapply pressure if bleeding is getting out of control.

⚠ Do not forget that a large sucker may be removing a large volume of blood from the patient while keeping your operating field dry!

- If you still cannot get control consider dividing the iliac artery overlying the bleeding point to access the vein—the artery is easier to repair than the vein.
- Once you have seen the bleeding point, try and lift it up between forceps and place a side-biting clamp (e.g. small Satinsky) around the defect. Use a continuous 5/0 or 6/0 Prolene suture to close the defect. If you can see only one end of a tear, control the rest of the bleeding site with direct pressure from a swab on a spongeholder and start suturing closed the end of the tear you can see—the rest will gradually come into view as you progress, moving the pressure swab along the tear as you go. Try to avoid picking up the vein wall opposite the defect so that you maintain patency.
- If a venous tear cannot be repaired despite the above manoeuvres, the bail out move is to pack the pelvis to control the bleeding and send the patient to ITU for overnight support and correction of any clotting deficiencies that will have developed with high volume transfusion. Return the next day with adequate experienced help when it is usually possible to repair the vein, although with a high chance of pelvic vein thrombosis.

Managing femoral vein bleeding
- This again presents as welling up of a large amount of dark blood in the wound.
- Apply direct compression.
- Inform anaesthetist of blood loss, place head-down, and resuscitate with IV fluids.

- Follow principles above for iliac vein bleeding. Access should be easier. Enlarge incision if necessary to ensure adequate access.
- If a clear view of the bleeding point cannot be achieved, place direct pressure on common femoral vein over the area of bleeding and divide the deep fascia to expose more of the vein above and below this point.

Aortic surgery

Abdominal aortic aneurysm

Background

- The abdominal (infrarenal) aorta is considered aneurysmal at $\geq$ 3cm in AP diameter.
- Most aortic aneurysms are fusiform in shape and arise below the renal arteries.
- Most aneurysms are asymptomatic until rupture and thus are diagnosed as incidental findings in the elective setting.
- There is a strong case for population screening with ultrasound in males over 60y where there is a 5% incidence.

Aetiology and natural history

- Aneurysmal dilatation of the aorta results from a degenerative condition of the arterial wall resulting in local dilatation.
- The recognized risk factors for aneurysm formation are male sex, positive family history, hypertension, and smoking.
- The natural history of aortic aneurysms is to continue to expand at an increasing rate until rupture or death from other causes.
- Less commonly, they may present with ischaemia from occlusion or distal embolization.
- Inflammatory aneurysms (< 5%) may be painful and cause local obstructive (ureteric or intestinal) symptoms.

Management

- Smoking cessation; control hypertension and other atherosclerotic risk factors.
- Ultrasound surveillance to monitor size.
- Open or endovascular repair, preferably electively.

Elective surgery

- Indicated to prevent rupture.
- Open tube graft repair is the gold standard treatment and is of proven durability but carries a mortality rate of 5%.
- Endovascular repair is in a stage of technical development. It has a lower initial mortality than open repair but requires lifelong monitoring and frequent re-intervention (usually radiological). Long-term durability not yet established.
- Aneurysms below 5.5cm in AP diameter have a low risk of rupture and should continue in surveillance.[1]
- At 5.5cm the annual risk of rupture is 5% and increases exponentially with continued expansion of the aneurysm. Elective repair is indicated for fit patients with aneurysms of diameters of 5.5cm or greater.
- In unfit patients the risk of surgical mortality has to be balanced against the risk of rupture without surgery.

Aneurysm imaging

- Ultrasound measurement of the AP diameter is most accurate modality for determining size.
- CT is superior for determining the relationship of the aneurysm to the renal arteries and detecting anomalies such as retro-aortic left renal vein or horseshoe kidney. It is important in assessing patients' suitability for endovascular repair (see p. 248). It may also identify concomitant intraabdominal pathologies such as colorectal cancer.
- CT may overestimate aneurysm size by 5–10% compared with ultrasound.
- Angiography visualizes only the vessel lumen so is not useful for imaging aneurysms which are usually partially filled with thrombus.

Clinical assessment

- History should include arterial risk factors, other coexistent arterial disease, respiratory dysfunction, medications, and previous surgery.
- Examination is aimed at identifying cardiac and respiratory disease but should also include palpation of the aneurysm, noting any tenderness and looking for abdominal scars, colostomy sites, etc. The femoral and distal lower limb pulses should be palpated and their presence and any aneurysmal expansion (commonest in femoral and popliteal arteries) noted.

Predicting operative risk

- Advanced age, cardiac disease, renal impairment, and respiratory dysfunction are the major predictors of adverse outcome. These and other variables can be used to stratify risk formally with scoring systems. The most common causes of perioperative mortality are MI and multi-organ failure.
- The Glasgow aneurysm score, Possum, and APACHE systems have been validated to predict mortality for open aneurysm repair (see boxes).
- Cardiac function is routinely assessed preoperatively with exercise echocardiography or radioisotope scanning to determine the presence of correctable inducible ischaemia. Patients with significant coronary disease should undergo revascularization prior to aortic surgery (Chapter 7).

Alternative approaches

- Open repair of aneurysm with tube or bifurcated graft (aorto-iliac or aortobifemoral).
- Stent graft of aorta and a variable part of the iliac system.

The precise extent of open repair or stent grafting depends on the extent of aneurysmal involvement.

Glasgow aneurysm score

Calculated using the formula:

  Risk score = age in years + the following:

- 17 points for shock
- 7 points for myocardial disease
- 10 points for cerebrovascular disease
- 14 points for renal disease

where
- myocardial disease refers to previously documented MI, or ongoing angina pectoris, or both
- cerebrovascular disease comprises all grades of stroke including TIA
- renal disease is defined as s serum level of urea > 20mmol/L, a serum level of creatinine > 150mmol/L at the time of surgery, a history of chronic or acute renal failure or a combination of these.

Scores > 77 have higher mortality in elective patients[1]

The physiological and operative severity score for the enumeration of mortality and morbidity (POSSUM)

Physiology score
- Age
- Cardiac signs
- Respiratory signs
- Systolic blood pressure
- Pulse rate
- Glasgow Coma Score
- Serum urea
- Serum sodium
- Serum potassium
- Haemoglobin level
- White blood cell count
- ECG result

Operative score
- Grade of operation
- Number of procedures
- Total blood loss
- Peritoneal soiling
- Presence of malignancy
- Timing of operation

Acute physiology and chronic health evaluation (APACHE) score

APACHE score = physiology score + GCS points + age points + chronic health score

Physiology score
- Temperature
- Blood pressure
- Heart rate
- Respiratory rate
- PaO_2
- pH
- $SerNa^+$
- K^+
- Creatinine
- HCT
- WCC

Chronic health points
- Liver cirrhosis
- Angina
- Chronic airways disease
- Renal failure
- Immunocompromised

Aorto-iliac occlusive disease

- Most likely to produce significant stenosis (> 50% diameter reduction) in iliac arteries.
- Affects aorta particularly at and beyond renal arteries.
- May be significant renal ischaemia in association with aortic disease.
- May produce erectile impotence.
- Needs correcting before more distal revascularization of the legs.
- Usually caused by atherosclerosis but consider:
  - post-irradiation accelerated localized atherosclerosis;
  - fibromuscular dysplasia;
  - Takayasu's disease.

Imaging

- Arterial duplex (limited by calcification, obesity, abdominal distension).
- Transfemoral angiography—access not possible if both iliac systems heavily diseased or occluded; can be combined with angioplasty/stenting.
- CT angiography—high contrast load. Therefore use caution if renal function impaired.
- MR angiography—unlikely to give clear images if aortic or iliac stents in situ.

Treatment options

- Balloon angioplasty ± stenting.
- Aortofemoral bypass graft.
- Iliofemoral bypass graft.
- Femoro-femoral cross-over graft (see Chapter 19).
- Balloon angioplasty + femoro-femoral cross-over graft (see Chapter 19).
- Axillo-femoral bypass graft (see Chapter 19).

Surgery for aorto-iliac aneurysmal and occlusive disease

Preoperative investigations (elective surgery)

- Recent measurement of aneurysm size and relationship to renal arteries.
- CT angiogram if endovascular repair.
- FBC.
- U & E, creatinine.
- Prothrombin time.
- Cross-match 2–4 units blood depending on size of procedure.
- Serum albumin if concerns regarding patient's nutrition.
- CXR (? thoracic aneurysm, lung disease, CCF).
- ECG.
- Stress echocardiogram.
- Respiratory function tests (spirometry) if there is any suggestion in the history or examination of COPD.
- If not previously checked measure blood glucose and serum cholesterol.

Main operative risks

- Myocardial ischaemia associated with aortic cross-clamp.
- Renal failure if aortic clamp has to be suprarenal for a juxtarenal aneurysm or if there is a period of significant hypotension associated with bleeding or unclamping of the aorta (shouldn't happen with a good anaesthetist and communication between surgical and anaesthetic teams).
- Bleeding from the anastomoses, particularly if local endarterectomy is required, leaving a fragile arterial wall.
- Left colon ischaemia if collateral blood flow from superior mesenteric artery via marginal artery is compromised (inferior mesenteric artery will be sacrificed during the surgery although is often already occluded) and flow to inferior rectal arteries impaired because of failure to maintain good flow to the internal iliac arteries. Usually only one internal iliac artery is required to maintain good pelvic perfusion but pre-existing disease in one of the iliacs may make it critical to reperfuse the other one.
- Iliac vein bleeding. The iliac veins lie behind the iliac arteries and may be stuck to them. Great care must be taken in freeing up the iliac arteries to sling them (see Chapter 12). Iliac veins bleed profusely and access is difficult.
- Ureteric damage. The ureters cross the iliac bifurcations. Take great care when isolating and clamping the external and internal iliac arteries that the ureters are not damaged—identify and sling out of your way.

Operative details See following sections.

Postoperative care—first 24 hours

- Routinely monitor in ITU/HDU for ~12h.
- Epidural anaesthesia continued.

- IV fluids, blood transfusion, insulin, inotropes, oxygen, and respiratory support are administered as required.
- Routine blood tests—FBC, prothrombin time, aPTT, U & E, creatinine, arterial blood gases.

Monitoring for potential complications during the first 24h post-surgery

Cardiac ischaemia
- ECG: ischaemia, arrhythmias.
- Mean arterial pressure low.
- CVP high.
- Serum troponin ↑.

Respiratory compromise (collapse, infection, left ventricular failure, ARDS post-transfusion)
- Respiratory rate ↑.
- Oxygen saturation low.

Renal (ATN, renal embolization)
- Urine output ↓.
- Creatinine rising.

Abdomen (bleeding, intestinal ischaemia)
- Distension.
- Oozing from wound.
- Abdominal compartment syndrome (increased intra-abdominal tension associated with reduced urine output).
- Tender over left colon.
- Rectal bleeding.

Legs (ischaemia, compartment syndrome, spinal cord damage)
- Leg pulses.
- Foot colour and temperature.
- Ankle/brachial pressure indices reduced or Doppler signal unobtainable.
- Muscle tenderness and increased compartmental tension.
- Lower limb neurological deficit (may be difficult to decide whether related to epidural or spinal ischaemia).

Management of early postoperative complications
- Leg ischaemia (trash foot)—embolectomy (see Chapter 14).
- Leg compartment syndrome (only occurs with reperfusion in acute severe leg ischaemia)—urgent fasciotomies under LA on ITU if necessary.
- Haemorrhage (low BP and CVP, abdominal distension, and falling Hb). Correct any coagulopathy with warming and clotting factors and re-explore early if evidence of continued bleeding.
- Renal failure. Adequate fluid filling; then loop diuretic. If hyperkalaemic, IV calcium gluconate or insulin/dextrose infusion; haemofiltration (and subsequent haemodialysis) may be necessary.

- Myocardial ischaemia: anticoagulation with heparin if no evidence of intraabdominal bleeding 24h post-surgery. tPA cannot be used with recent surgery.
- Respiratory failure: physiotherapy, antibiotics, diuretics, and ventilation as appropriate.
- Intestinal ischaemia: diagnosed on flexible sigmoidoscopy, CT scan. Managed conservatively if only mild tenderness and little bleeding but, if suspect full thickness significant wall ischaemia, perform a Hartmann's procedure before colonic perforation and uncontrolled graft contamination.
- Paraplegia. An uncommon (< 0.7% aortic aneurysm surgery) but devastating complication. Diagnosis using MRI spinal cord. Steroids may reduce associated oedema and functional deficit but otherwise conservative management.

Postoperative care after 24h
- Continue epidural analgesia for 2–3 days.
- Restore normal diet within 48h if tolerated.
- Mobilize.
- Chest physiotherapy.
- Check bloods day 1 and 2.
- Remove catheters and lines day 1/day2.
- Discharge when fit after day 3.

Complications after 24h
- As for early postoperative complications, although bleeding becomes less likely after 24h.
- Mural haematoma of 4th part of duodenum may present with upper abdominal discomfort due to gastric distension, and vomiting about a week post-surgery after the patient has been eating satisfactorily for a few days. Management is NG drainage, IV fluids, and wait for resolution (occasionally TPN required).

Long-term complications
- Aneurysmal expansion above graft.
- Graft infection through contamination at operation or superficial infection in the groin wound that spreads to affect the graft.
- Development of false aneurysm at either anastomosis (with open surgery).
- Aorto-intestinal fistula may present 15–20 years after open surgery. Most often seen with bifurcated aortic grafts, perhaps because of bowing forward of the graft as it lacks the restraint of a more proximal anastomosis (see p. 238).
- Aortic stent grafts may develop an endoleak, fracture a stent, or migrate distally.

Elective tube graft for aortic aneurysm[*]

Indication

Aneurysm affecting only the aorta, i.e. without extension into the iliac arteries, that has reached a size when the risk of rupture or embolization outweighs the risk of surgery.

Anaesthesia, preparation, and draping

- GA with epidural analgesia.
- Arterial line, CVP line, and peripheral access are inserted for monitoring and fluid and drug administration.
- A urinary catheter is inserted and connected to an hourly urimeter bag.
- Expose and shave the abdomen from nipples to mid-thigh allowing extension of incision along length of abdomen and access to the femoral arteries.
- Skin is prepared with povidone–iodine or chlorhexidine.
- The surgeon usually operates from the patient's right side.
- Broad-spectrum prophylactic antibiotics are administered.
- NG tube is not routinely required.

Incision and approach

- Transabdominal (vertical or transverse incision); **or**
- Retroperitoneal (oblique incision; see Chapter 12, p. 194).

Procedure

1 Expose the neck of the aneurysm, usually below the renal arteries (see Chapter 12). Dissect out the origins of the common iliac arteries to allow application of vertical clamps. There is danger of injury to the common iliac veins during this dissection.
2 Give IV heparin (70IU/kg) and allow to circulate for 2min before the application of clamps.
3 DeBakey or Fogarty clamps are applied to the common iliac artery origins.
4 An aortic clamp is applied to the aneurysm neck while pulling down the aneurysm with the right hand. Adequate clamping is confirmed by loss of aortic pulsation.
5 If the inferior mesenteric artery is identified at the anterior surface it may be oversewn with 3/0 Prolene.
6 The aortic sac is opened longitudinally with an 11 blade and Mayo scissors. The organized thrombus that normally occupies the aneurysm sac is scooped out. A self-retaining retractor (Norfolk and Norwich) is inserted into the aneurysm to display its internal wall.
7 Blood and thrombus are removed with suction and swabs.
8 Rapidly move on to arrest back-bleeding from lumbar vessels by oversewing the orifices with 3/0 Prolene in a vertical plane, facilitated by grasping the bleeding orifice with an Alliss clamp.

[*] OPCS code L19.4.

9 Extend the arteriotomy to the top of the aneurysm. Carry the incision laterally for a centimetre around each side to display the neck to which the graft will be sutured. The iliac orifices are displayed similarly at the distal end (Fig. 13.1).

10 The tube graft (usually Dacron, 18–24mm) is selected based on estimate of the neck size.

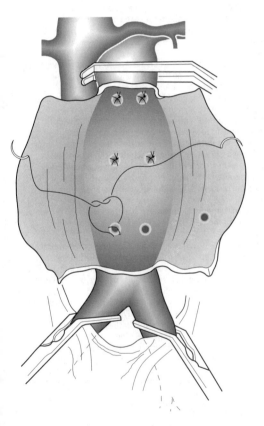

Fig. 13.1 Opening the aortic sac to display aortic aneurysm neck and aortic bifurcation for anastomoses.

11 Before suturing the top end anastomosis, cover the distal clamps with a damp pack to avoid catching the suture in their ends.

12 Use a full-length double-ended 2/0 or 3/0 Prolene suture (preferably 120cm long) on a round-bodied needle. For the first stitch pass the needle from outside to in, in the posterior midline of the graft, pull through to midsuture length, and then pass vertically in a cranial caudal direction, picking up the aortic wall on the posterior midline of the aortic neck where there is often a useful ridge (Fig. 13.2).

13 Continue with a parachute technique across the back wall of the anastomosis then tighten the sutures and proceed with a continuous suture round on each side to reach the midline anteriorly. Reverse the final stitch so that the two suture ends are tied across the anastomosis.

14 The integrity of the anastomosis is tested by clamping the graft and releasing the top end clamp. Reclamp and repair any points of significant bleeding (see p. 236).

15 Pull the graft out under gentle tension to reach the iliac orifices and trim any excess graft beyond this point.

16 Wash the iliac orifices and tube graft out thoroughly with heparinized saline to remove any thrombus or debris.

17 Anastomose the distal graft to the edge of the common iliac artery origins using a 3/0 suture and a parachute technique initially, completing with a continuous suture that is tied across the anastomosis anteriorly, as at the proximal anastomosis. Wash out the graft and distal orifices with heparinized saline before completion.

18 Warn the anaesthetist of impending clamp release.

19 Release one of the iliac clamps to check the integrity of the anastomosis.

20 The limbs are reperfused sequentially. Compress the femoral artery below the iliac clamp you have already removed and then remove the aortic clamp. This will sweep any debris into the internal iliac circulation where hopefully it will do less damage than down the femoral artery. After about 15sec remove compression from the groin. There will probably be a moderate drop in BP and a rise in expired CO_2 if the limb has satisfactorily reperfused. Wait for the anaesthetist to bring systolic pressure back above 100mmHg before repeating the procedure on the other side.

21 When there is satisfactory haemostasis, use continuous 2/0 Vicryl to close the aortic sac and then the peritoneum over the graft, making sure that it is completely covered. The abdomen is closed with continuous 0 nylon (in layers if transverse or oblique incision) and the skin with subcuticular Monocryl.

22 The feet are inspected for signs of ischaemia before removing the drapes and unscrubbing. If either foot is cold and mottled or white without pulses (especially if there is an obvious difference between the feet) consider proceeding directly to a femoral embolectomy (see p. 316) to remove debris that has usually been dislodged from the aortic sac.

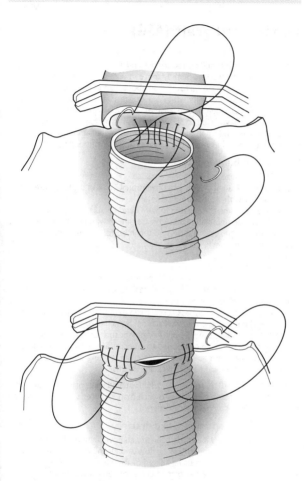

Fig. 13.2 Inlay technique for aortic graft anastomosis.

Aortic stent graft (ASG)[*]

Indications

Aneurysm of the aorta and/or iliac arteries under the following circumstances.

- Where aorta measures 5.5cm or more in widest AP diameter or isolated iliac aneurysms greater than about 4cm diameter.
- The lower initial mortality with ASG[2] suggests it might be indicated in patients who are high risk because of cardiac or respiratory disease but trials to date have failed to show a survival advantage in this group.[3]
- In the 'hostile' abdomen due to retroperitoneal inflammation, scarring, etc., which would increase the difficulty and risk of open repair.

Patient suitability for ASG

- Aortic, aorto-iliac, or iliac aneurysms.
- Use either CT angiography or conventional CT and digital subtraction angiography with a measuring catheter.
- Not all aneurysms are suitable for ASG and each graft manufacturer has criteria for suitability. Detailed assessment with regard to diameter, angulation, shape, calcification, and thrombus is required of:
  - the proximal neck;
  - the distal landing zones;
  - the access vessels.
- Where parameters are exceeded there is a price to pay in terms of the ease of deployment and risk of endoleak (pressurization of the aortic aneurysm sac that may lead to rupture).
- The use of adjunctive bypass surgery can extend the role of ASG, by allowing the stent to cover vital arterial branches to provide a satisfactory landing zone. Leading edge fenestration and branch technologies are being developed to incorporate renal and/or visceral arteries to make possible the endovascular stenting of more extensive juxtarenal and thoraco-abdominal aneurysms.

Preoperative work up See p. 236. Detailed measurements of aorta/iliac arteries are made according to each manufacturer's instructions. The suitable device components are ordered.

Anaesthesia, preparation, and draping

- Aortic stent grafting should be done in an environment that has operating theatre standards of air flow and cleanliness—either in the angio suite or in theatre using a fixed or mobile C arm.
- The procedure can be performed under regional anaesthesia.
- The patient is placed supine on an X-ray table. The monitoring and other preparation is the same as for an open tube repair. Draping needs to extend beyond the feet. This helps ensure a sterile area for the angio wires and introduction of the device components.

---

[*] OPCS codes: L28.1, aortic; L28.5, aortic-iliac.

Procedure

See Fig. 13.3.

1   The femoral arteries are exposed and controlled in each groin.
     (A totally or partially percutaneous technique is possible using
     remote suture closure devices.)
2   Systemic heparin 5000IU is given.
3   The femoral arteries are punctured and a sheath placed in each groin.
4   Under image intensifier control an ultrastiff wire is negotiated from
     the right femoral through the iliac system and aneurysm all the way
     around the aortic arch to sit in the ascending aorta.
5   A pigtail catheter is advanced up the left side to the level of L1.
6   An angiogram is taken to show the renal arteries down to the
     internal iliac arteries.
7   If there is marked iliac tortuosity, a measuring catheter may be
     introduced up the right side to recheck the distance from the aortic
     neck to the landing zone in the iliac. The act of placing the stiff wire
     changes the configuration of the iliacs, tending to straighten them
     out. If available or anticipated the option of a choice of limb
     extensions may then be exercised.
8   The main body device is prepared by flushing with heparinized saline
     and introduced up the right side. A formal arteriotomy is not
     required; the artery simply splits horizontally as the device sheath is
     introduced. The body is orientated while screening observing the
     manufacturer's radio-opaque markers.

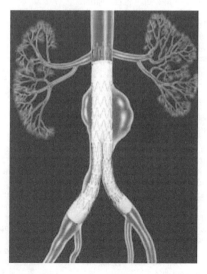

Fig. 13.3 Aortic stent graft in place.

9   An angiogram centred and magnified on the renal arteries is performed. Most aneurysms angle forwards at the proximal neck. The extent can be determined on the planning CT scans. The C arm is angled craniocaudally to take this into account.

10 Using landmarking, road mapping, or most simply a dry marker on the X-ray monitor, the level of the renal artery orifices is noted.

11 The position of the patient and C arm are held while deploying the body of the device while screening. Just prior to deployment the pigtail catheter is withdrawn to prevent it catching in the uncovered portion of the stent graft.

12 The C arm is repositioned to show the iliac landing zones.

13 An angiogram demonstrates the position of the internal iliac arteries.

14 Poor opacification of the right external iliac is due to the large sheath virtually occluding the femoral artery. A combination of information from the earlier run and the better shown contralateral side is used to accurately place the limb extension.

15 The right limb extension is deployed. Ensure a minimum two zig overlap with the body component and leave the internal iliac in circulation. Where there is no suitable landing zone in one common iliac the internal iliac orifice is covered on that side. Some prefer to embolize the internal iliac up front to prevent an endoleak. If there is no suitable landing zone in either common iliac, some cover both internal iliacs accepting the risk of buttock claudication. Using branched stent technology one internal may be stented with a suitable device to keep it in circulation.

16 The contralateral short limb of the body is cannulated from the left groin. The use of angled or specially shaped catheters and Terumo ultraslippery guide wires facilitate this. It is important to understand the configuration of the body component, e.g. the position of the short limb lies anterior to the long limb rather than side to side for some manufacturers. Hand injection of contrast confirms successful cannulation of the short limb. The stiff wire may then be transferred to the left side and advanced through the stent graft and around the arch of the aorta.

17 The left limb is deployed in a similar manner to the right side.

18 The top end, component joins, and distal landing zones are moulded with the special balloon.

19 A check angiogram is taken looking for endoleaks and satisfactory deployment.

20 Minor type II leaks can be accepted in anticipation that they will thrombose spontaneously by the 1 month check CT scan.

21 Type I endoleaks need to be dealt with. Further ballooning may cure the problem. If the top end has not sealed a stent extension or uncovered stent may be deployed.

22 The sheaths are removed from the groins as clamps are applied and the femoral arteries repaired with a 5/0 polypropylene suture. Care is taken to ensure the intima and outer layers are sutured together so as not to risk a dissection flap. The feet are checked after clamps have been released.

Postoperative care Patients do not require high dependency following the procedure, and a hospital stay of only 2–3 days is required in most cases.

Follow-up and monitoring

Patients require follow-up monitoring indefinitely to exclude endoleak.

Endoleaks

- Type I. Around the proximal or distal landing zones of the device
- Type II. From native branches of the aneurysm sac that have failed to thrombose
- Type III. Through the joins between the various modular components of the graft or through a tear in the fabric of the graft
- Type IV. Porosity through the graft leading to endotension with expansion of the sac of the aneurysm

There are currently no clear indications as to which endoleaks require intervention and which can continue to be monitored. Adjunctive information regarding shrinkage of the aortic sac or pressure measurements may inform which endoleaks should be treated. Generally types I and III require correction. Most endoleaks can be dealt with endovascularly either by extension grafts or thrombosing the vessel causing a type II endoleak.

Open aortic surgery for ruptured aortic aneurysm

Indications

When there are clinical or radiological grounds for making the diagnosis of ruptured AAA in a patient likely to survive surgery with a reasonable life expectancy and who wishes to go ahead with surgery.

- Clinical grounds. Acute onset of hypotension ('feeling faint', collapse, or losing consciousness) associated with lumbar back pain and sometimes mid or lower abdominal pain. BP and conscious level often improve, although BP usually fails to reach normal for the patient (which is often in the hypertensive range). On examination a pulsatile abdominal mass. If no mass palpable then ultrasound is usually the quickest way of establishing the diagnosis of AAA (but cannot confirm rupture).
- Where clinical grounds for diagnosis are less clear cut and the patient appears stable, the CT angiogram will confirm/exclude rupture. CT without contrast may support the diagnosis with what appears to be haematoma adjacent to the aorta and oedema but this is not definitive.

The apparently stable patient can decompensate at any time and delay in CT scan may mean the difference between surviving surgery and dying. It is routine therefore to operate on clinical grounds in most patients, CT being used mainly to reassure and pursue alternative management in the patient in whom the diagnosis is in serious doubt.

A patient who remains unconscious from hypotension due to ruptured AAA is very unlikely to survive surgery in more than a vegetative state and should be managed conservatively.

Alternative approaches

- Endovascular aortic stenting is performed in a few centres with the expertise and available implant stock to perform the operation as an emergency in a patient stable enough to allow aortic CT imaging and with favourable anatomy (i.e. negotiable iliac arteries and adequate infrarenal neck).
- Conservative management in the patient unlikely to survive or unwilling to undergo surgery. Usually patients die within 12h. Occasionally a rupture is sufficiently contained to stabilize in which case the patient is often asymptomatic and does not require admission, although at some stage they are likely to suddenly destabilize and die from their rupture.

Preoperative investigations

- Send urgent bloods for FBC, U & E, PT, and 8 unit cross-match but do not delay transfer to theatre until results are available.
- In patients with collapse, back pain, and vomiting (unusual in ruptured AAA) send serum amylase to exclude pancreatitis.
- Baseline ECG to check for evidence of myocardial ischaemia.

* OPCS codes: L18.4, aortic tube graft; L18.6, bifurcated graft.

Anaesthesia, preparation, and draping
- Patient supine.
- Central and peripheral lines are placed, the abdomen and groins shaved, and urinary catheter inserted, but no anaesthesia is given until the patient is prepared and draped and the surgeon is ready to start the operation. Relaxation of the abdominal muscles may remove tamponade from the aorta and allow increased bleeding so the time from anaesthesia to control of bleeding needs to be minimized.
- Prepare the abdomen from above the xiphisternum to pubis and down to and including both groins. Drape to expose these areas. A large adhesive operative site drape is useful to hold the drapes in place around the pubis and groins.
- Broad-spectrum prophylactic antibiotics.
- GA without epidural.

Incision and approach The aim must be to gain access to the aortic neck and place a clamp to control bleeding as quickly as possible without causing significant damage to intervening structures. Thereafter the pace of the operation can slow down to normal. Make a midline incision from xiphisternum to just above the pubis using the blade rather than scissors for speed but being careful to avoid adherent bowel.

Operative steps
1   Move small bowel over to right of midline to expose the aorta and confirm the diagnosis of rupture from the bulging haematoma surrounding the aorta (patients who have freely ruptured into the peritoneal cavity are unlikely to survive long enough to make the operating table unless it occurs after they arrive in theatre).
2   Landmarks may be distorted by haematoma but try and find the 4th part of the duodenum as this will be approximately the level where you need to place the aortic clamp, assuming the aneurysm is infrarenal. Incise the peritoneum around the 4th part of duodenum and mobilze it towards the right to allow access to the underlying aorta. Dissect with scissors down on to the aorta at this point and, if aneurysmal, follow it up and backwards on to the neck. Once the neck is identified clear 2–3cm length, then free each side down on to the spine, using mainly blunt dissection with the forefinger but avoid tearing any lumbar arteries. It is usually possible to clear sufficient space to place an aortic clamp on the neck without disrupting branches. If it proves impossible to locate the aneurysm neck rapidly, consider achieving control by placing an aortic clamp temporarily at the diaphragm (see p. 192) where the anatomy should be clear.
3   Turn your attention to the iliac arteries, which should be palpable through the peritoneum. Decide whether they are aneurysmal (they may even be the site of rupture) and therefore whether your repair will be with a tube or bifurcated graft. A bifurcated graft requires significantly longer aortic cross-clamp time and therefore imposes a greater stress on the heart than a tube graft. If the patient is elderly it is reasonable to leave small iliac aneurysms alone.

4 If planning a tube graft proceed as on p. 240, but do not give heparin. If planning a bifurcated graft because of aneurysmal common or internal iliac arteries proceed as on p. 252 and again do not give heparin.

5 Ask your anaesthetist to check clotting and platelets once you have control and are putting the graft in. It is very likely that FFP and possibly platelets will be needed. Get these ordered as soon as possible so that they can be given soon after the clamps are released and you are reasonably certain that the anastomoses are secure.

Postoperative care After repair of a ruptured aneurysm patients are at high risk of all the complications listed on pp. 237–8. Their coagulation is probably still abnormal so have it checked again once the patient reaches ICU and correct accordingly.

Aorto-iliac bypass graft*

Indication Aortic aneurysm extending into common iliac arteries or in association with separate common iliac aneurysm(s). The graft is taken down to the common iliac bifurcation or on to the external iliac artery (which is never aneurysmal).

Aorto-iliac bypass grafting takes significantly longer aortic cross-clamp time than an aortic tube graft. In a patient in whom, because of age or other co-morbidity, you would prefer to keep the cross-clamp time short and whose life expectancy (and iliac aneurysm growth time) is limited, it may be better to ignore a small common iliac aneurysm (< 3cm) or gather up the dilated neck of a common iliac artery on to the end of an aortic tube graft.

Anaesthesia, preparation, and draping
- GA with epidural.
- Patient supine.
- Urinary catheter.
- Expose, shave, and paint the abdomen with antiseptic from xiphisternum to pubis. Do the same to both groins in case surgery has to be extended to the groin.
- Drape around these areas with adhesive transparent film to anchor drapes in place.

Incision and approach Transabdominal approach gives access from the infrarenal aorta to the external iliac artery. Best access is via a vertical (midline) incision but in a short wide abdomen an infraumbilical transverse incision also gives adequate exposure (see Chapter 12).

Procedure
See Fig. 13.4.
1 Isolate neck of aortic aneurysm (see Chapter 12).
2 Isolate and sling external ilac artery preferably just beyond its origin (for a distal anastomosis at the iliac bifurcation), but if this is difficult because of dense adhesions (e.g. inflammatory AAA) or access around a large common iliac aneurysm then isolate it close to the inguinal ligament.
3 If planning anastomosis at the iliac bifurcation, lift up on the external iliac sling to expose and sling the origin of the internal iliac artery. If the internal iliac artery is aneurysmal, you will have to consider excluding it but, if both internal iliac arteries are aneurysmal, it is probably sensible to keep the smaller one in circulation to ensure a good pelvic blood supply. If an internal iliac aneurysm is to be excluded, follow it down into the pelvis to find and sling its major branches.
4 Give heparin IV (70u/kg).
5 Place clamps on external and internal ilac arteries (if iliac bifurcation not dissected then clamp across aneurysmal common iliac artery (CIA)).

* OPCS code L19.6.

6 Place clamp on aortic neck of aneurysm, preferably below the renal arteries but if inadequate space between renal arteries and aneurysm, clamp will have to be placed suprarenally and upper anastomosis completed securely in as short a time as possible.

7 Open aortic sac longitudinally, evacuate fresh clot and laminated thrombus to expose lumbar arteries (posterior) and inferior mesenteric artery (anterior), if patent. Oversew back-bleeding lumbar and inferior mesenteric arteries with 2/0 Prolene.

8 Wash out distal end of aortic neck with saline and decide on aortic bifurcated graft size from this (the iliac limb size does not matter). Shorten body of graft to 2–3cm length.

9 Anastomose the graft starting posteriorly in the midline, using a parachute technique for the first three sutures on each side and 2/0 or 3/0 Prolene (preferably 120cm long), positioning the graft within the aortic neck (inlay technique).

10 Place your hand or a clamp across the graft just below the anastomosis. Warn the anaesthetist that there may be some blood loss while you test the anastomosis by removing the upper clamp. Inspect both front and back of the anastomosis.

11 If your aortic clamp was suprarenal move it down to the graft 2–3cm below the anastomosis.

12 Move your retractors if necessary to expose the iliac arteries on one side.

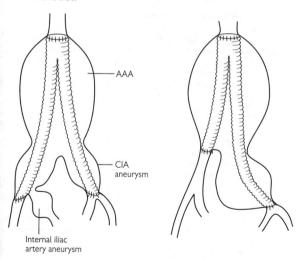

AAA

CIA aneurysm

Internal iliac artery aneurysm

Fig. 13.4 Possible sites for distal anastomoses of aorto-iliac bypass graft.

If planning to anastomose to the iliac bifurcation

13a Open the CIA longitudinally, extending into the first 0.5cm of external iliac artery. On the right this can be the full length of CIA but on the left the nervi erigentes cross the common iliac artery and need to be preserved if possible. Dissect them free first or open only the distal common iliac artery/first 0.5cm external iliac artery.

14a Pull the graft down through the aortic sac, taking the appropriate iliac limb down through the CIA under gentle tension and divide it obliquely so that the shorter posterior wall reaches the proposed anastomosis line, which runs around the origins of both the internal and external iliac arteries, and the oblique cut edge matches the anastomosis line in length (Fig. 13.5).

15a Use 3/0 or 4/0 Prolene for this distal anastomosis, starting in the midline posteriorly with a parachute technique and laying the graft within the distal vessels.

16a Once suturing is complete remove the internal and external iliac clamps to allow back bleeding and check the security of your anastomosis.

17a When happy with your anastomosis get your assistant to apply firm pressure over the femoral artery on that side, apply a clamp to the other limb of the graft close to its origin, and remove the aortic clamp. Any debris will be swept into the internal iliac circulation. After about 15sec release the femoral artery compression.

If planning to anastomose to the external iliac artery

13b Place two slings on the artery either side of your planned anastomosis (approximately 2cm apart) and clamp outside the slings.

14b Make a longitudinal arteriotomy in the anterior wall approximately 1.25cm long. Flush out the opened artery with saline to remove any clot or other loose debris.

15b Cut the appropriate limb of the graft to length, taking it retroperitoneally anterior to the iliac vessel under gentle tension and fashioning an oblique end to match your arteriotomy. Use 3/0 or 4/0 Prolene to construct an end-to-side anastomosis.

16b Tie off the external iliac artery above your anastomosis. Clamp the other (unanastomosed) limb of the graft just below its origin and release the aortic clamp.

17b You still have a common iliac clamp in place. If the internal iliac artery is not obviously aneurysmal then tie or sew off (depending on size) the CIA near its origin—it will thrombose down to its bifurcation without needing to expose the latter. If the internal iliac artery is aneurysmal you will need to assess whether it is worth the risk of obliterating it. If there are dense adhesions and a small iliac aneurysm it may be best left. If the internal iliac branches have been isolated then tying them off external to the aneurysm is relatively straightforward. If you cannot get to the branches then the aneurysm can be opened and the back-bleeding origins of the branches oversewn, but this will inevitably lead to blood loss, which may be significant (Fig. 13.6).

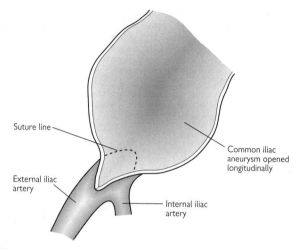

Fig. 13.5 Preparation of anastomosis site at common iliac bifurcation.

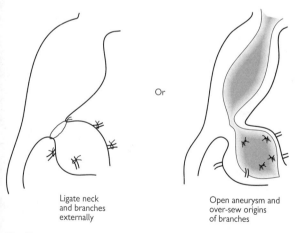

Fig. 13.6 Dealing with an internal iliac artery aneurysm.

Final steps

18 Repeat the procedure on the other side. If the common iliac artery is normal on one side the iliac limb of the graft on this side can be anastomosed to the common iliac origin in an inlay fashion with 3/0 or 4/0 Prolene (in such a case it is probably best to perform the anastomosis on this side first because the procedure is quicker and the aorta can be unclamped earlier).

19 Once happy with haemostasis, close artery over the graft where possible with 2/0 Vicryl and complete coverage of the graft by closing the peritoneum with 2/0 Vicryl. Close the abdominal wall.

Aorto-bifemoral bypass graft[*]

Indication Occlusive disease affecting the infrarenal aorta and/or both iliac arteries. Even if the external iliac arteries are open, they are likely to be diseased and to stenose or occlude in the future so an aorto-iliac graft should be avoided.

Anaesthesia, preparation, and draping

- Patient supine.
- GA with epidural.
- Arterial line, CVP line, and peripheral access are inserted for monitoring and fluid and drug administration.
- Urinary catheter with a urimeter so that urine output can be measured on a regular basis.
- IV broad-spectrum prophylactic antibiotics.
- Expose, shave, and paint with antiseptic the abdomen from nipples to pubis and down over each groin to the upper thigh.
- Drape to expose abdomen from xiphisternum to pubis and down to each groin, securing the drapes with clear plastic adhesive film.

Incision and approach

- Transabdominal—vertical midline from just below xiphisternum to 3cm above the pubis or transverse either just above or below the umbilicus or
- Retroperitoneal—via an oblique incision (see Chapter 12).

Procedure

1 Expose the aorta for 4–5cm below the renal vein as in Chapter 12. Sling the aorta at each end of your exposure.
2 Expose both common femoral arteries and origins of SFA and profunda (see Chapter 12). Sling CFA just below inguinal ligament and SFA and profunda at their origins.
3 Make a retroperitoneal tunnel from the aortic exposure to each groin by passing a curved aortic clamp up from the groin, under the inguinal ligament, following the posterior curve of the iliac vessels up to the aorta. Grasp a tape or long silastic sling with the clamp and draw it back down through the tunnel to mark its position. Clip the two ends of tape or silastic sling together. It is important to do this before giving heparin.
4 Give 70IU/kg heparin IV and wait 2min for it to circulate.
5 Clamp each end of the exposed aorta.
6 The aortic anastomosis can be end-to-end or end-to-side. If there is a large inferior mesenteric artery (which has often developed as a collateral pathway with occlusive iliac disease) then it is probably sensible to keep it in circuit by performing an end-to-side aortic-graft anastomosis. Otherwise the decision lies with the surgeon's preference.

[*] OPCS code L19.6.

End-to-end anastomosis

7a Divide the aorta transversely and completely about 1cm below upper clamp.

8a Oversew distal end of aorta with 2/0 Prolene. Remove lower clamp and check haemostasis here.

9a Select aortic bifurcated graft based on size of proximal aorta. Cut body of graft to about 2cm length with a transverse cut. Use 2/0 (120cm) or 3/0 continuous Prolene to perform your anastomosis, starting in the midline posteriorly with a parachute technique for the first six sutures and laying the edge of the graft within the aorta (Fig. 13.7).

10a Once the anastomosis is secure, pinch the graft or clamp it closed and release the aortic clamp (having warned your anaesthetist first!) to test the suture line. Lift up the graft to check it posteriorly. Reclamp and repair any points of significant bleeding (see Chapter 12).

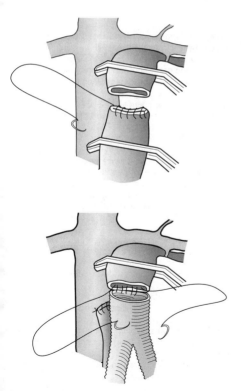

Fig. 13.7 End-to-end aortic graft anastomosis.

End-to-side anastomosis

7b Make a longitudinal incision of approximately 3cm in a relatively soft part of the anterior aortic wall between the clamps. Wash out the exposed interior of the aorta.

8b Select a bifurcated graft approximately the same size as the exposed aorta. Cut obliquely across the body of the graft, shortening it to about 3cm on its longest anterior wall and 2cm on its posterior wall (Fig. 13.8).

9b Anastomose the end of the graft to the arteriotomy, starting at the heel of the graft, joining it to the lowest part of the arteriotomy with 2/0 (120cm) or 3/0 Prolene and continuing round to the front with a continuous suture.

10b Once the anastomosis is finished, pinch or clamp the graft and release the top clamp (having warned your anaesthetist!) to test your suture line. Reclamp and repair any sites of significant bleeding (see Chapter 12).

Final steps

11 Separate the two ends of tape/silastic sling, attach the curved aortic clamp to the end emerging in the groin, and pull the clamp up through the tunnel with the other end. Detach the tape/sling and attach the clamp to the end of the appropriate graft limb, making sure that it is not twisted. Cover the abdominal wound with damp packs and turn your attention to the groin.

12 Clamp the CFA at the inguinal ligament and the SFA and profunda artery at their origins. Make a longitudinal arteriotomy about 1.5cm long in the anterior wall of the CFA. If the SFA is occluded so that profunda provides the only run-off, it is sometimes useful to skew the arteriotomy slightly so that it runs into the origin of profunda and so that any origin stenosis is widened when the graft hood is sewn in place. Pull the graft down into the groin firmly but gently so that the limbs are under slight tension and cut the end of the graft obliquely to create a hood that runs anteriorly. Use 4/0 continuous Prolene suture to anastomose graft to arteriotomy, starting with the heel/top of arteriotomy and a parachute technique.

13 Warn the anaesthetist that you are about to reperfuse a leg. Clamp the unanastomosed graft limb just below its origin; release the profunda clamp in the groin and the aortic clamp. After about 10–15sec unclamp the SFA. The BP will fall (even with an extremely good anaesthetist) and expired CO_2 rise if the limb is successfully perfused. The anastomosis should have no more than a slight ooze of blood, which will stop. If there is significant bleeding you will have to reclamp and repair the anastomosis.

14 Repeat the procedure in the other groin.

15 Check all operative areas for haemostasis. Once dry, close the peritoneum over the aorta and graft with 2/0 Vicryl and each groin with two layers of 2/0 Vicryl (deep fascia and Scarpa's fascia) and an absorbable subcuticular skin suture.

16 Before removing the drapes ask theatre staff to expose both feet to
    check that they are pinker than before. If the clinical improvement
    does not match what was expected from the preoperative arterial
    assessment (e.g. palpable foot pulses if SFA and crural vessels are
    patent) then assess run-in to the groin (is there a good pulse in the
    graft limb, if necessary measuring femoral pressure with a needle on
    a manometer line provided by the anaesthetist?). Poor run-in can be
    caused by thrombus in the limb of the graft, twisting or kinking of
    the graft, or compression in its tunnel, especially at the inguinal
    ligament. Thrombus can be cleared with a no. 6 Fogarty catheter
    passed up through a transverse incision in the graft hood in the
    groin. Twisting and kinking may require taking down the distal
    anastomosis, untwisting or straightening the graft, and refashioning
    the distal anastomosis, if necessary, with an extension of graft
    material in order to align the new hood with the arteriotomy. Any
    constricting bands, including the lower fibres of the inguinal ligament,
    should be divided. If run-in looks good then consider passing an
    embolectomy catheter (no. 4 Fogarty) down SFA and profunda to
    retrieve any debris that may have been dislodged. Foot perfusion will
    also be affected by the degree to which the patient is well filled
    and, if CVP and BP are low, the foot will tend to be cooler and
    paler and pulses more difficult to feel.

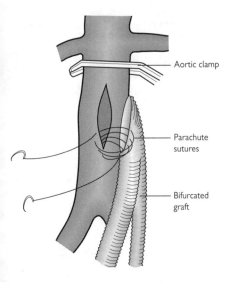

Fig. 13.8 End-to-side aortic graft anastomosis.

Surgery for suprarenal aortic aneurysms

Large aortic aneurysms sometimes extend proximally to involve the renal arteries; occasionally the SMA and coeliac axis are involved. A thoraco-abdominal aneurysm extends a variable distance down the abdominal aorta and may involve mesenteric and renal arteries.

Preoperative imaging to confirm the proximal extent of an aneurysm is important in elective repair so that the risks of intervention, inevitably higher with involvement of renal arteries, SMA, and coeliac axis, can be judged and balanced against the risk of rupture and the surgery can be planned appropriately. CT or MR angiography are usually required to assess the proximal extent if routine vascular ultrasound does not clearly show that the aneurysm is infrarenal.

Options for intervention

- Open repair with aortic graft and re-implantation of visceral arteries.
- If the aneurysm extends just above one or both renal arteries it is usually possible to cut the aneurysm neck obliquely so that the renal artery origin(s) remain attached to the proximal aorta. This may require clamping between or above the renal arteries until the proximal anastomosis is complete. The surgery is otherwise the same as for infrarenal aneurysm repair.
- Endovascular repair is under development with fenestrated grafts placed as for infrarenal aneurysms but extended up to the suprarenal neck. Fenestrations are secured over visceral branches with stents extending out into the branch.

Open repair of suprarenal aortic aneurysm with re-implantation of visceral arteries[*]

Indication

- Aneurysm that has reached a size where the risks of rupture outweigh the risks of surgery. There are little data on the risk of rupture with increasing size in the suprarenal region, but a minimum size of 6.5cm is probably reasonable.
- A patient with ruptured suprarenal aneurysm is unlikely to survive surgery if the SMA and coeliac axis are involved.

Preoperative work up As for infrarenal aneurysm but with imaging of proximal extent as above.

Anaesthesia, preparation, and draping

- GA.
- Patient supine with upper torso rotated to left with left arm supported over body with armrest, pelvis horizontal.
- Broad-spectrum prophylactic antibiotics IV.
- Urinary catheter.
- Shave and prepare skin from left mid-thorax to groins.
- Drape to expose left lower thorax, abdomen, and groins.

Incision and approach

- Thoraco-abdominal incision through distal half of 9th or 10th intercostal space and extending obliquely across abdomen to the midline; then down towards the umbilicus (Fig. 13.9).
- Retroperitoneal approach to reach the neck of the aneurysm, both renal arteries, and SMA and coeliac axis, by mobilizing left colon, spleen, tail of pancreas, and left kidney over to the right (Fig. 13.10). The diaphragm is cut in a radial direction for several cm to improve access and the crus of the diaphragm may need dividing to reach the neck.

[*] OPCS codes L19.3 + L41.3.

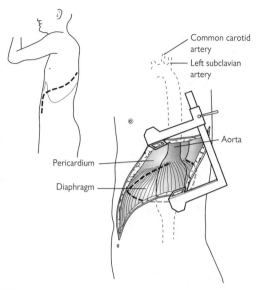

Fig. 13.9 Incision for access to suprarenal aorta.

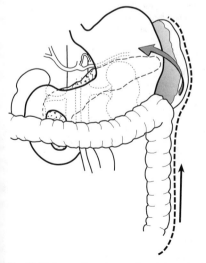

Fig. 13.10 Retroperitoneal approach to abdominal aorta.

Procedure

1 Isolate the neck of the aneurysm sufficiently to allow clamping at a later stage. The visceral branches do not need to be dissected out.
2 Dissect out the common iliac arteries (access to the right can be improved by dividing the inferior mesenteric artery and extending the incision across the midline if necessary). If the infrarenal aorta is of normal calibre the dissection can be performed at this level instead.
3 Place clamps on the aortic neck and both common iliac arteries or lower aorta. Heparin is not needed prior to this. Surgery now needs to move rapidly to minimize visceral ischaemia time, preferably keeping it less than 30min.
4 Make a longitudinal incision in the aneurysm sac passing behind the left renal artery (Fig. 13.11) up to the neck. Extend the incision transversely around the distal edge of the neck for 1–2cm each side to improve access.
5 Anastomose an appropriate sized Dacron graft in an inlay fashion to the neck of the aneurysm with 2/0 Prolene. Check for haemostasis around the suture line.
6 Cut out a patch from the aneurysm bearing the coeliac axis, SMA, and right renal artery origins and a separate patch with the left renal artery origin. Alternatively cut a single patch bearing all 4 vessels if the intervening aortic wall is not grossly expanded and thinned. Anastomose these to appropriately placed fenestrations made in the graft with 5/0 Prolene (Fig. 13.12).
7 Move the aortic clamp down to the Dacron graft below the re-implantation sites and release the slings to allow reperfusion.
8 Complete the surgery with a distal anastomosis to the normal lower aorta or the aortic bifurcation as for an infrarenal aneurysm repair (p. 240).
9 Put in chest drain prior to wound closure.

Complications of surgery

As for infrarenal aortic surgery but with ↑ mortality (published mortality rates are about 10%), ↑ risk of renal failure, and ↑ respiratory problems because of thoracotomy.

In addition:
• risk of ischaemic damage to fore- and midgut structures;
• risk of paraplegia due to possible exclusion of artery of Adamkiewicz from circulation.

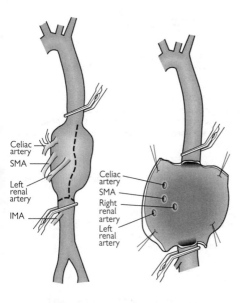

Fig 13.11 Opening suprarenal aneurysm behind left renal artery.

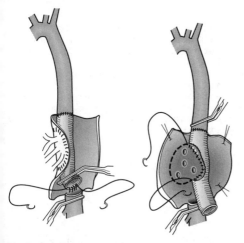

Fig 13.12 Anastomosing renal and visceral artery origins to graft.

Ilio-femoral bypass graft[*]

Indications
- Occlusive disease of the ipsilateral distal iliac system.
- Occlusive disease of the contralateral iliac system (ilio-femoral cross-over graft).

Anaesthesia, preparation, and draping
- Warn the anaesthetist that, although the surgery and clamping may be confined to one iliac arterial system, it is quite common to need more proximal clamping on the aorta (e.g. because occlusive disease more extensive than expected).
- Patient supine.
- GA or epidural.
- Arterial line, CVP line, and peripheral access for monitoring and fluid and drug administration.
- Urinary catheter.
- IV broad-spectrum prophylactic antibiotics.
- Expose, shave, and paint with antiseptic the abdomen from nipples to pubis and down over each groin to the upper thigh.
- Drape to expose abdomen from xiphisternum to pubis and down to groins.

Incisions and approach
- Iliac artery:
  - curved iliac fossa incision for an extraperitoneal approach *or*
  - midline vertical incision for a transperitoneal approach.
- Femoral artery. Curved or vertical groin incision (see Chapter 12).

Procedure
1 Expose the CIA (see Chapter 12) and, if possible, mobilize sufficiently to place slings 3cm apart. If rigid and difficult to separate from underlying iliac vein then clear sufficiently to place a vertical clamp on each side of the anastomosis site.
2 Expose and sling the CFA at the inguinal ligament and the origins of the SFA and profunda artery.
3 Create a retroperitoneal tunnel from the exposed iliac artery down to the groin, passing deep to the inguinal ligament. If performing an ilio-femoral cross-over graft this will need to run in the retroperitoneal space across the pelvis to the opposite inguinal ligament and groin.
4 Give heparin 70u/kg IV.
5 Lay a 6 or 8mm reinforced PTFE graft in the tunnel.

---

[*] OPCS codes: L50.6, emergency; L51.6, elective.

6   Clamp the iliac artery either side of the anastomosis site. Make a longitudinal arteriotomy and check run-in. It is common to need a local endarterectomy because of atheromatous flaps or stenosis. If necessary extend the arteriotomy proximally to a clamp at the common iliac origin to allow an extensive endarterectomy. If this is insufficient you will need to consider the aorta, the other CIA, the other femoral artery, or even the axillary artery as an alternative source of inflow.

7   Create an end-to-side or end-to-end anastomosis between PTFE and common iliac artery using 3/0 Prolene or PTFE suture. Clamp just beyond the anastomosis and remove the proximal clamp. The PTFE will ooze from stitch holes so wrap in a gauze swab until haemostasis is achieved.

8   Clamp the groin arteries and perform an end-to-side anastomosis between the PTFE graft and the common femoral artery, if necessary with a local endarterectomy. If the SFA is occluded then take the arteriotomy into the proximal profunda artery so that the graft effectively widens the profunda origin to ensure good run off. Release clamps and wait for haemostasis, if necessary reversing the heparin with protamine.

9   Close the abdominal incision in muscle layers with an absorbable suture and the skin with a subcuticular absorbable suture. Close the groin with two layers of Vicryl and the skin as above.

Iliac endarterectomy*

Indication for surgery Occlusive disease of the iliac artery.

Anaesthesia, preparation, and draping
- Patient supine.
- GA with epidural.
- Arterial line, CVP line, and peripheral access for monitoring and fluid and drug administration.
- Urinary catheter.
- IV broad-spectrum prophylactic antibiotics.
- Expose, shave, and paint with antiseptic the abdomen from nipples to pubis and down over each groin to the upper thigh.
- Drape to expose abdomen from xiphisternum to pubis and down to groins, securing drape with clear plastic adhesive film.

Incision and approach Make a curved incision in the iliac fossa for an extraperitoneal approach or a midline incision for a transabdominal approach.

Procedure
1 Dissect out the common and/or external iliac artery for the extent of the disease and a cm or two beyond each end (watch out for the ureter crossing the iliac bifurcation). If the disease involves the origin of the internal iliac artery then place a sling around its origin.
2 Give 70u/kg heparin IV.
3 Clamp the iliac arteries above and below the imaged/palpable disease. Make a longitudinal arteriotomy along the anterior wall of the artery between the clamps.
4 Perform an endarterectomy to remove atheromatous plaque narrowing the lumen. Make sure the distal edge of intima beyond the endarterectomy is securely adherent. If it is tending to lift (test by squirting heparin saline on to it) then secure it with interrupted 6/0 sutures. Wash out any debris in the lumen.
5 Close the arteriotomy with a patch—usually synthetic but vein (LSV from the groin) can be used if anxious to avoid synthetic material.
6 If a transabdominal approach has been used then close the peritoneum over the artery with continuous 2/0 Vicryl.
7 Standard closure of the abdominal wall.

---

* OPCS code L52.1 (with patch).

Treatment of aorto-enteric fistula[*]

The aorto-enteric fistula (a connection between lumen of aorta and lumen of bowel) occurs most often at the top end of an aorto-bi-iliac or bifemoral bypass graft and is thought to develop from erosion of the suture knot through the wall of the bowel (usually 4th part of duodenum) followed by development of an abscess between the two structures that then erodes into the aorta. Rarely, an ungrafted aortic aneurysm will also erode into adherent bowel to produce a fistula.

It presents with GI bleeding, often 1 or 2 'herald' bleeds producing haematemesis followed by a catastrophic 'bleed out' that the patient is unlikely to survive. If the diagnosis can be made before the terminal bleed then the condition may be treatable, at least in the short term.

Diagnosis
- Clinical suspicion. Upper GI bleeding in the presence of an aortic graft (often put in a few years previously), sometimes slightly raised temperature, raised inflammatory markers (WBC, ESR, CRP).
- Oesophagogastroduodenoscopy reveals no cause for bleeding above 4th part of duodenum and inflammation and adherent blood clot in 4th part of duodenum (if reached).
- CT scan shows fluid and gas collection around/adjacent to aorta/aortic graft and close apposition of bowel loop to aorta.

Possible treatments
- Excision of top end of graft and replacement with new (perhaps silver-impregnated or rifampicin-soaked) graft.
- Excision of entire graft and replacement with axillo-bifemoral bypass graft.
- Excision of entire graft and replacement with vein panel graft (using superficial femoral vein).
- Conservative management (± antibiotics) in those patients who are unlikely to survive any major surgery, accepting that they are likely to die from this complication in the near future but improving their general condition by suppression of sepsis.

The synthetic graft is inevitably bathed in pus and the purist approach is to remove it all, but that involves major surgery for perhaps a frail patient and is not guaranteed to eliminate infection or prolong life—the new graft may become infected and the aortic stump may 'blow'. Removal of only grossly contaminated graft material and any pus, replacement with fresh graft material, and then long-term antibiotic treatment based on the microbiology of the excised graft material are more likely to produce at least short- to medium-term patient survival.

---

* OPCS codes: L22.3, local replacement; L22.4 + L16.2, excision and replacement with axillo-femoral graft; L22.4 + L20.4, excision and replacement with autologous vein.

Preparation for surgery

- This is an emergency situation and, although all surgical options involve aortic clamping (sometimes above the renal arteries), there is no time for complex cardiac work up to optimize the patient so the assessment of their operative risk has to be done on clinical grounds + ECG.
- Baseline bloods for U & E, creatinine, FBC, ESR, CRP, and cross-match 6 units blood.
- Avoid antibiotic treatment before surgery and do not give 'prophylactic antibiotics' until samples for microbiology are retrieved from the region of the fistula. Then give broad-spectrum antibiotics, following advice from the microbiology department, until the responsible organism is identified.
- If planning an axillo-bifemoral bypass graft decide which axillary artery is preferred (on the basis of arm pressures, siting of colostomies, or scarring that might interfere with tunnelling of graft from chest to groin) and warn the anaesthetist to use the other arm for their arterial line.
- If planning a vein panelled graft obtain a venous duplex of both legs to check that there is a good profunda system to provide alternative venous drainage.

Local replacement of infected graft

See Fig. 13.13.

1   GA. Patient supine with abdomen and groins prepared (just in case you need access to the femoral arteries, e.g. for a femoral embolectomy) and urinary catheter in place.

2   Midline incision through old scar and transperitoneal approach to the aorta (you cannot repair the bowel via a retroperitoneal approach). You will usually find the 4th part of duodenum densely adherent to the aorta with surrounding inflammation, often an abscess cavity full of pus and loops of adherent small bowel.

3   Approach the aorta above the inflammatory mass, below the pancreas to try and place a controlling clamp. This may have to be above the renal vein (and renal arteries). If it proves impossible to do safely, consider placing a temporary clamp on the aorta at diaphragm level (p. 192) to gain control, moving the clamp down as soon as the lower aorta becomes visible with clearance of the adherent bowel. Place another aortic clamp on the graft below the inflammatory mass. Peel the inflammatory mass off the aorta/aortic graft (take it off as a whole rather than peeling off individual loops of bowel—you need to work reasonably fast if clamped above the renal arteries). Put a bowel clamp over the bowel to control leakage from the fistula point.

4   Often you find the upper anastomosis completely disrupted. Take what is left of it down and trim the aortic stump back to firm tissue that will hold sutures. Send samples for microbiology and give a dose of broad-spectrum antibiotics. Take some fresh graft of the same size (silver-impregnated or rifampicin-soaked may be preferable) and anastomose it to the aortic stump with 2/0 or 3/0 Prolene.

5   Trim the infected old graft back (it is not uncommon to find a relatively long body left in these cases) taking off as much of the grossly contaminated graft as possible down to just above the bifurcation. Trim back the new graft so that the old and new grafts can be anastomosed end-to-end with 2/0 or 3/0 Prolene without any slackness that would allow the new composite body to bow forward and might lead to another fistula.

6   Repair the defect in the bowel with one or two layers of absorbable suture.

7   Wash out the area of the fistula with dilute Betadine.

8   Mobilize a tongue of greater omentum so that it lies across the two new lines of aortic graft anastomosis to separate it from overlying bowel (in particular the 4th part of duodenum). Tack the omentum in place.

9   Standard closure of the abdominal wall.

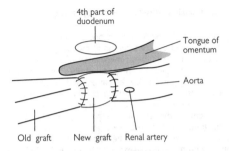

Fig. 13.13 Local replacement of an infected aortic graft. Lateral view of aorta showing omental strip used to separate anastomotic sites from duodenum.

Replacement with axillo-bifemoral bypass graft

See Fig. 13.14.

The operation can be performed in one session with removal of the infected graft followed by axillo-bifemoral bypass grafting. This offers at least the theoretical advantage of minimizing infection of the new graft (the patient is re-prepped and draped between removal and replacement), but it is a long procedure for patient and theatre team and once started there is usually no option to delay the second part because of complications, as the legs are unlikely to survive. The alternative is to put in the axillo-bifemoral bypass graft first, possibly the day before removal of the aortic graft. There is probably a greater risk of infection because antibiotics are not given until after the aortic graft is exposed.

1   If starting with the axillo-bifemoral graft, follow details in Chapter 19. In the groins a new (more distal) anastomosis site (e.g. SFA in midthigh) needs to be selected if the previous graft came down to the common femoral arteries. Ensure that the new anastomosis site is kept separate from and uncontaminated by the original groin anastomosis site. If the graft is intra-abdominal anastomose the new graft to the common femoral arteries. You may wish to tie off the artery above this point to prevent competitive flow from the old graft that might lead to new graft thrombosis. Close and dress the wounds carefully with adherent film dressing to seal them and prevent contamination.

2   Then proceed (same or following day) with removal of the aortic graft. Make a midline incision and follow steps 1–3 in 'Local replacement of infected graft', p. 274. Send samples for microbiology and give a dose of broad-spectrum antibiotics. Close the aortic stump with two layers of 2/0 Prolene or a bowel stapling device oversewn with 2/0 Prolene.

3   Peel the graft down and mobilize the two limbs (if bifurcated) as far as the inguinal ligament or any more proximal anastomosis point. If an aorto-bifemoral graft, ligate and divide the graft at the inguinal ligament. If the distal anastomoses are intra-abdominal, clamp the vessels and take down the anastomoses. The arteries will need ligating or repairing with a vein patch depending on the quality of the vessel.

4   Close the bowel end of the fistula with a single or double layer of absorbable suture and wash out the contaminated bed of the graft with dilute Betadine. Mobilize a tongue of greater omentum and tack it down to the bed of the graft, covering the aortic stump to prevent bowel adhering. Close the abdominal wound and seal with adherent plastic film.

5   If there are groin anastomoses to take down proceed with these. The graft remnants can then be pulled out from under the inguinal ligaments. Close the common femoral arteriotomy with a vein patch. Close the groin wound and seal with adherent plastic film to prevent contamination of the new anastomosis sites.

Replacement with autologous vein

1 Harvest superficial femoral vein from both legs and store in
   heparinized saline. Close the leg wounds.
2 Remove the aortic graft as above.
3 Fashion a new aortic graft using each superfical femoral vein's limb
   and bringing them together proximally to create a new graft body
   that is then anastomosed to the aortic stump. Anastomose the distal
   limbs of the new graft to the same sites as the previous graft.

Postoperative assessment monitoring See pp. 237–8.

Main risks

- Disruption of aortic stump with catastrophic bleeding.
- Infection of new graft.
- Renal failure (sepsis and suprarenal clamp).
- Graft occlusion leading to leg ischaemia.
- Distal embolization leading to multiple infected areas or leg ischaemia.
- Pelvic ischaemia (mainly left colon) if axillo-bifemoral graft with CFA
  proximal ligation.

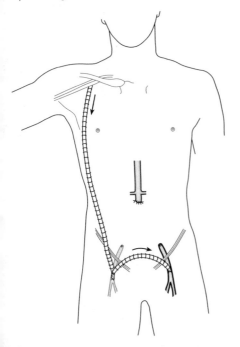

Fig. 13.14 Replacement of infected aortic graft with axillo-bifemoral graft.

References

1. The UK Small Aneurysm Trial Participants (1998). Mortality results for randomised controlled trial of early elective surgery or ultrasonographic surveillance for small abdominal aortic aneurysms. *Lancet* **352** (9141), 1649–55.
2. EVAR Trial participants (2005). Endovascular aneurysm repair versus open repair in patients with abdominal aortic aneurysm (EVAR trial 1): randomised controlled trial. *Lancet* **365** (9478), 2179–86.
3. EVAR Trial participants (2005). Endovascular aneurysm repair and outcome in patients unfit for open repair of abdominal aortic aneurysm (EVAR trial 2): randomised controlled trial. *Lancet* **365** (9478), 2187–92.

Infrainguinal revascularization

Infrainguinal revascularization for chronic ischaemia

- Common femoral endarterectomy and femoro-popliteal bypass graft to the popliteal artery above the knee are relatively straightforward, low-risk procedures.
- As surgery extends below the knee, with smaller run-off vessels, longer bypass grafts, and more time-consuming and demanding surgery, the risks of intervention increase.
- Grafts passing below the knee are generally reserved for patients with ischaemic rest pain or tissue loss.
- The more proximal procedures are performed in patients with claudication that has failed to respond to non-operative measures, as well as those patients with rest pain or tissue loss.
- Common femoral endarterectomy is often combined with femoro-popliteal or femoro-distal bypass grafts to provide adequate inflow.
- Atherosclerosis is a generalized disease and, if a patient has extensive disease in the leg (requiring a long bypass graft), the heart and brain are also likely to have extensive disease. This is reflected in the much higher mortality with femoro-distal bypass graft (10%) than with above- or below-knee femoro-popliteal bypass graft (2–5%).

Alternatives to surgery

- Conservative management of claudication (see Chapter 5) and dressings, analgesia, antibiotics as necessary.
- Balloon angioplasty (including subintimal PTA) of diseased vessels can sometimes be performed down to ankle level if necessary . There is decreasing success with length of disease and distance down leg and occasionally technical failure precipitates further thrombosis and possibly leg loss. The overall risk to the patient is significantly less than with surgery which is usually still an option if PTA fails.
- SFA occlusive disease can sometimes be managed with acceptable results with overlapping 6mm covered stents. Bare stainless steel stents have not been shown to be superior to angioplasty in clinical trials but nitonol stents are superior to angioplasty in long segment disease. Covered stents have some theoretical advantages over bare stents but the first randomized controlled trial, the VIBRANT trial, is not due to report until 2008. Long segment > 10cm stenosis and occlusions can be treated providing there is a least one good run-off vessel and the
  patient takes dual antiplatelet agents. The lesion needs to be crossed first, either luminally or subintimally, and predilated with angioplasty prior to deploying the stent(s). Covered stents can also be used as a bail-out procedure for complications of angioplasty, such as intimal flaps and dissections or unsatisfactory dilatation due to recoil or calcified lesions.
- Phenol lumbar sympathectomy may improve tissue perfusion in rest pain and help ulcer healing if tissue loss is small (p. 76).

Clinical assessment

- History should include inquiry into arterial risk factors, other arterial disease, respiratory dysfunction, medications, allergies, and previous surgery.
- Examination is aimed at identifying cardiac and respiratory disease and assessing the site of disease and severity of ischaemia in *both* lower limbs (the other leg is often not far behind in disease severity).
    - Record all palpable pulses. A good external iliac artery pulse should be palpable just above the groin, even if the CFA is occluded, at least in a slim patient.
    - Check sensation. Ulceration may have more to do with a peripheral neuropathy than vascular disease.
    - Measure the ABPI on both sides.

Adequate inflow and run-off for the graft

- Grafts must have good run-in and outflow to stay patent. This can usually be decided on the preoperative arterial imaging (duplex or angiography).
- If preoperative imaging leaves some doubt about inflow or run-off, fall back plans need to be made and the patient warned that the surgery may be more extensive than initially planned. Preparation for surgery needs to take this into account (e.g. alerting the radiologists and theatre staff to the possible requirement for an on-table angioplasty, exposing the other groin for a femoro-femoral bypass graft, exposing the lower leg for a more distal bypass graft).
- Adequate run-in is usually confirmed by releasing the clamp to ensure there is 'audible' flow.
- Adequate run-off can be tested by heparin saline injection using a syringe to test for distal resistance but if there is any doubt do an 'on-table' angiogram.
- There is no point in putting in a bypass graft when inflow or run-off is inadequate. If you suspect this preoperatively, but are not sure, then discuss with the patient with severe ischaemia the option of proceeding to an amputation under the same anaesthetic if exploration reveals inflow or run-off inadequate to sustain a graft.

Preoperative investigations

- Arteriogram (TFA or CTA) or arterial duplex to show arteries from infrarenal aorta to foot (dependent duplex may pick up patent distal arteries missed by angiography).
- Vein mapping. If the GSV, preferably in the affected leg is clearly present and greater than 4mm in diameter over sufficient length for the bypass graft, it needs marking with the patient standing. If it is not clearly seen then vein mapping with duplex becomes necessary. If neither GSV is adequate, check the LSVs (although shorter) and the superficial veins of the arm (cephalic and basilic). If arm veins are likely to be used then guard them against venepuncture by writing 'NO NEEDLES' in large letters on arm.

- Retrieve reports on any ulcer or other swabs taken recently to determine whether MRSA is present because it will influence antibiotic prophylaxis
- Foot X-ray if there is ulceration to look for osteomyelitis which may be an indication for foot surgery at the same time as bypass grafting. If there is a high clinical suspicion and foot X-ray is negative then MRI is useful.
- Routine cardiac assessment by clinical assessment and ECG (stress echo, etc. not usually required). A patient with poor cardiac function is unlikely to sustain flow through a long distal bypass graft even if they survive the 4–8h surgery it may require.
- Respiratory function. Clinical assessment should include the patient's ability to lie flat (or at least on no more than three pillows) because, although the risks of surgery in patients with poor respiratory function can be reduced with the use of epidural, the patient still has to be comfortable lying flat enough to allow groin access (assuming the graft runs from the CFA).
- Baseline bloods: U & E, FBC, and cross-match 2 units blood.

Instruments and equipment
- Ensure angiography available and suitable operating table in use.
- Doppler with sterile transducer (sterile laparoscopy bag).
- Grafts available in case required.
- Embolectomy catheters.

'On-table' angiography
- Use an umbilical catheter (size 6F) when imaging the run-off from an arteriotomy.
- Use a 21G 'butterfly' needle with a clamp proximally if checking flow in a closed artery or graft.
- Flush initially with heparin saline to ensure there is no leak and that injection is possible (you do not want the operative field obscured on X-ray by leaking contrast medium).
- Position the C arm over the injection site.
- Ensure that all personnel in theatre (including the surgeon) have adequate lead protection.
- Prepare a 10mL syringe with 50:50 Niopam (or similar)/saline mix
- Inject a small amount while imaging with the C arm.
- Repeat a sequence of images down the leg to give a complete picture of runoff as far as the foot. Limit total volume injected to 15mL.
- Look for narrowing of the graft lumen, suggesting twisting or external compression, thrombus/debris within the graft, distal anastomotic hood, or run-off.
- Flush the catheter or needle with 10mL heparin saline to wash out the contrast. If a needle has been used, place a 'z' stitch around the entry site, pull the ends up tight as the needle is removed, then tie to secure haemostasis when the proximal clamp is removed.

Strategies for dealing with poor flow through a graft

- If the graft is still pulsatile then get an 'on-table' angiogram from just below the proximal anastomosis.
- If the graft has thrombosed then open it transversely just above the distal hood and pass a no. 3 or 4 (depending on size of arteries) Fogarty embolectomy catheter proximally to clear the graft and restore good flow if possible. If the valves in a reversed vein graft prevent passage of the catheter you may have to open the graft transversely near the top anastomosis and flush the vein out with heparin saline. Pass the Fogarty catheter down across the distal anastomosis and into the run-off arteries as far as it will go to retrieve any debris or thrombus blocking run-off. Flush the distal arteries with heparin saline and, if there is resistance to flow, get an 'on-table' angiogram to determine the cause.
- Unless the run-off is poor there has to be a reason for failure of the graft to improve leg perfusion. Any of the following may apply:
  - twisting, kinking, and external compression of the graft;
  - a graft of inadequate length pulled too tight to reach the distal anastomosis;
  - poor technique causing outflow narrowing at the distal anastomosis;
  - a flap lifting in the outflow artery;
  - thrombus or atheromatous debris blocking graft or run-off;
  - using too small a vein;
  - missed tributaries or uncut valves in an in situ bypass graft;
  - inadequate anticoagulation;
  - heparin-induced platelet antibodies (HIT; p. 161).

Assessment at the end of surgery

- Are there distal pulses? If not, are they detectable on Doppler insonation? If not, can you detect a Doppler signal over the graft and how good is it? If graft flow is poor or undetectable with no evidence of distal flow, consider re-exploration before the patient leaves the table.
- Is the foot pink and warm? Any deterioration in colour may indicate graft failure but if the patient is underfilled or cold it may take a while for foot perfusion to improve despite a functioning graft.
- Is BP satisfactory? If low is there any evidence on ECG of myocardial ischaemia. If suspicious but not definitive, measure serum troponin. If no evidence of new myocardial ischaemia does patient need further filling to improve circulation?
- Check Hb. Over a long operation there may be unnoticed significant blood loss that elderly patients will not tolerate well. Transfuse early if HB low (< 9g/dL).

Postoperative instructions and management

- IV maintenance fluids and O_2 for 24h.
- Monitor pulse, BP, temperature, and O_2 saturation frequently in the first 24h.

- Monitor foot pulses by palpation or Doppler insonation and check foot colour hourly for the first 24h, then 4 hourly. Any deterioration needs to be reported promptly because a thrombosed vein graft can only be retrieved if re-opened within a few hours of thrombosis (the next morning is too late!).
- Measure ABPI bilaterally within 24h of surgery.
- If the graft is precarious (e.g. poor vein, thrombosed on table and had to be revised, patient with poor/unstable myocardial function) then consider full heparinization postoperatively unless you have already had significant bleeding problems. IV heparin is easier to control than sc LMWH if you run into problems with bleeding from the wounds postoperatively. Continue for 48h; then decide (perhaps on basis of duplex assessment of the graft) whether to discontinue or convert to warfarin.
- Arrange a duplex scan of the graft before discharge (may be too uncomfortable to do for a few days) and enroll in graft surveillance programme for 1 year.

Main risks

- Mortality rate 2–10% depending on length of graft; usually cardiac-related death.
- Myocardial infarction—see above.
- Graft occlusion and limb loss.
- Bleeding occasionally from groin anastomosis, often related to infection.
- Infection in groin or other wounds especially if distal ulceration provides a source.
- Postoperative leg oedema is common. Usually due to reperfusion of leg and lasts 1–2 weeks; occasionally due to DVT.

Table 14.1 1- and 5-year patency rates for infrainguinal bypass for critical ischaemia

	Primary (secondary) patency (%) at	
	1 year	5 years
Above-knee PTFE	76 (80)	48 (54)
Above-knee vein	83 (87)	69 (71)
Below-knee vein	84 (87)	68 (77)

Common femoral endarterectomy[*]

Indication and requirements

- Occlusion or tight stenosis of the femoral segment may give rise to symptoms and signs of limb ischaemia. This segment does not do well with balloon angioplasty or stenting due to the position of the inguinal ligament and the origin of the profunda femoris artery. Open surgery, by contrast, is straightfoward and and gives excellent results.
- Run-off to profunda at least is required. If the profunda artery is occluded at its origin but appears shortly below as good artery, then extension of the endarterectomy into profunda to remove the occlusion, and extension of the CFA patch into the origin to widen it, will probably maintain a good run-off.
- If the profunda artery is of poor quality then a femoro-popliteal bypass graft (assuming that the popliteal artery is patent) may be required at the same time to keep the CFA patent.
- Aside from whether the CFA will stay open, the question arises as to whether sufficient increase in blood flow will be achieved by CFA endarterectomy alone. If the patient has only claudication then it is probably all that is needed. A patient with critical ischaemia, however, usually requires correction of disease at two levels. Unless you have already angioplastied or bypassed aorto-iliac disease affecting this leg, it is unlikely that CFA endarterectomy alone will be sufficient. Where it is uncertain whether or not an infrainguinal bypass is required the proximal end of the GSV can be mobilized and utilized in the patch angioplasty while still in continuity so that a bypass can be performed at a later date by the in situ method without the need to re-enter the groin.

Anaesthesia, preparation, and draping

- GA, epidural, or even just LA infiltration are all options.
- Operating table suitable for X-ray screening of aorto-iliac vessels.
- Urinary catheter.
- Arterial lines and venous access for maintenance fluids, drugs, and transfusion if necessary.
- Broad-spectrum IV prophylactic antibiotics.
- Expose, shave, and prepare groin from above inguinal ligament to mid-thigh. If run-in is doubtful, prepare the other groin as well for a possible femoro-femoral cross-over graft and alert the radiologist that an on-table angioplasty may be required. If run-off is in doubt then prepare whole leg down to ankle and place foot in a transparent bowel bag in case a bypass graft is needed.

Incision and approach A vertical or oblique incision can be used (p. 198). There is no point in extending the incision above the inguinal ligament; disease in the distal EIA can be dealt with from the groin.

---

[*] OPCS codes: L60.1, + patch; L60.2, no patch.

Operative technique

1 Expose and control the CFA, SFA, and profunda artery. Follow the CFA cephalad, lifting up the inguinal ligament to expose the external iliac as far as is necessary to reach a disease-free segment of artery anteriorly. The atherosclerosis posteriorly in the artery often extends superiorly indefinitely and can be felt as a 'u' configuration. The superficial circumflex iliac and external pudendal arteries will be encountered at the level of the inguinal ligament and can either be divided and tied or controlled with a double sling of a n. 0 tie. Just above the level of the inguinal ligament the deep circumflex iliac vein crosses the artery and this should be tied in continuity and divided to avoid troublesome bleeding.

2 If a profundaplasty is planned the profunda is followed until it divides and its branches slung. The profunda vein crosses the artery near its origin and this needs to be carefully divided and tied to expose the profunda adequately.

3 Give 70u/kg heparin iv.

4 A baby Satinsky or spoon clamp is useful for the external iliac artery as this can be placed high on the accessible artery, beneath the inguinal ligament and clamped front to back, to avoid fracture of the atheromatous plaque, which can disrupt the arterial wall. Clamp the distal vessels.

5 Make a longitudinal arteriotomy in the CFA. If the start of disease is palpable then extend to just above this point; otherwise cut down the entire length of CFA. If run-off is via the profunda then angle the arteriotomy to run into the profunda, extending down until soft wall is encountered (Fig. 14.1).

6 A standard endarterectomy is performed within the CFA. If there is obvious inflow stenosis in the distal external iliac artery, the plaque can be mobilized circumferentially from below in the endarterectomy plane and pulled out with a Roberts or similar large clip, releasing the external iliac clamp as this is done. The plaque often fractures at the clamp and this marks the proximal extent of the endarterectomy. The Roberts clamp can be passed up several times to retrieve any further fragments of loosened plaque, easing the clamp on each occasion, until satisfactory inflow is achieved.

7 If inflow is still unsatisfactory the options are to proceed to an on-table angiogram with a view to an iliac angioplasty and/or stent or to proceed to a femoro-femoral cross-over graft.

8 Extend the endarterectomy if necessary, into the profunda artery. Great care must be taken to achieve a smooth end point; otherwise tacking sutures may be required.

9 Close the artery by direct closure with continuous Prolene suture (5/0) or by using a patch, depending on the size of the artery. The patch can be vein (anterior thigh vein or other good-sized tributary in the groin—if necessary the proximal end of the GSV), endarterectomized obliterated SFA divided and turned upwards, or prosthetic material (Dacron or PTFE).

10 In some cases it may be easier (and quicker) to simply replace the
common femoral artery from the level of the inguinal ligament to its
bifurcation or (if the SFA is occluded) to the profunda origin only.
The replacement may be vein, endarterectomized SFA, PTFE, or
Dacron.

Postoperative instructions
The patient can return to the ward and mobilize the following day. Home
in 2–3 days.

Follow-up
Special follow-up is not required.

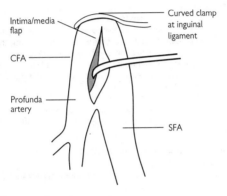

Fig. 14.1 Common femoral artery endarterectomy.

Femoro-popliteal bypass graft above knee*

Indication and requirements for surgery

- Critical ischaemia or calf claudication caused by occlusive disease of the superficial femoral artery.
- Surgery is generally reserved for cases in which conservative treatment has been maximized and angioplasty is not possible or has failed.
- There must be good run-in to the femoral artery.
- A patent above-knee popliteal artery and at least one continuous named vessel into the foot is the minimum run-off required.

Possible conduits

- Vein from the same leg, preferably GSV, is preferred by many. Usually the vein is reversed. The alternative is to use it 'in situ' with ligation of tributaries and division of valve cusps with a valvulotome, but this produces quite a severe angulation on the graft as it dives down from the surface of the leg to the popliteal artery, especially in a large leg.
- In the presence of open ulceration or distal infection it is important to avoid synthetic grafts if at all possible.
- In the absence of infection, some surgeons routinely use PTFE ('saving the vein for later use', quicker and easier). The 1 year patency rates for vein and PTFE in above-knee femoro-popliteal bypass grafts are similar (see Table 14.1, p. 285).

Anaesthesia, preparation, and draping

- GA or regional (epidural).
- Venous and arterial lines for drug administration, maintenance fluids, and transfusion.
- Urinary catheter.
- Broad-spectrum prophylactic antibiotics IV.
- Expose the lower abdomen above the groin and the leg down to ankle.
- Shave the groin and medial thigh and calf.
- Prepare and drape around the groin to above the inguinal ligament and the entire leg down to the proximal foot, placing the foot in a sterile transparent bowel bag.
- If the vein is to be harvested from the other leg, this will need to be prepared similarly.

Incision and approach The femoral vessels are exposed through a groin incision (p. 198). The above-knee popliteal artery is exposed through a medial thigh incision (p. 200). The GSV is harvested along its required length with or without skin bridges.

Procedure

1   Sling the CFA, SFA, and profunda artery. Confirm adequate inflow by palpating the common femoral pulse.

---

* OPCS codes. Elective: L59.2 (prosthetic); L59.3 (vein). Emergency: L58.2 (prosthetic); L58.3 (vein).

2 Sling the above-knee popliteal artery, preferably below any obvious disease. Take care when dissecting to avoid damage to the often adherent popliteal vein and tributaries.

3 Insert a 21G butterfly needle into the popliteal artery, clamp the artery above this point, and flush with heparin saline to check resistance to run-off. If there is any difficulty, place another clamp or double sling below the injection site and open the artery longitudinally at the puncture point to check for local disease. If necessary perform a local endarterectomy, extending the arteriotomy and endarterectomy distally until the artery opens up. If no suitable run-off point is found despite extending popliteal exploration down towards the knee joint, consider proceeding to a below-knee bypass graft.

4 Once the length required for the bypass graft (to the distal end of the popliteal arteriotomy) is established then harvest vein or cut a length of 8mm PTFE (if using vein in situ, see p. 300).

5 Use a tunneller to create a tunnel deep to sartorius muscle in the groin, bringing it out deep to muscle in the lower incision. Lay the graft (reversed if vein) in the tunnel.

6 Give 70u/kg heparin iv.

7 Clamp the groin arteries and make a longitudinal arteriotomy in the CFA approximately 12mm long, avoiding obvious plaque if possible. Wash out the exposed lumen with heparin saline. Check inflow by releasing the CFA clamp for a second or so. If inflow is poor it may be improved by local endarterectomy in the proximal CFA/distal EIA (see p. 286). If this fails to produce 'audible' inflow, either on-table iliac artery angioplasty or femoro-femoral cross-over graft will be necessary before proceeding with the infrainguinal graft.

8 Spatulate the proximal end of the graft and anastomose end-to-side to the CFA using 4/0 or 5/0 Prolene (or PTFE if using PTFE graft).

9 Clamp the graft close to the anastomosis (you do not want blood sitting and clotting in a synthetic graft prior to establishing flow in it) and release the arterial clamps. If there is significant anastomotic bleeding reclamp and repair.

10 Make a 10mm longitudinal arteriotomy in the popliteal artery (unless already opened) and flush with heparin saline.

11 Cut the graft to length (pulled straight but not tight) and cut to length to reach the distal end of the anastomosis. Create a hood on the end of the graft. If an extensive arteriotomy has been required to achieve good outflow, consider closing the proximal part of it with a vein patch so that the hood of the graft does not need to be excessively long.

12 Anastomose the graft end to side to the popliteal artery using 5/0 Prolene. Before placing the last two sutures, release the proximal clamp on the graft to flush out the graft.

13 Release the proximal popliteal clamp (to divert any residual debris away from the distal leg) and unclamp the graft. After a few seconds, release the distal popliteal clamp.

14 Feel for popliteal and pedal pulses; check colour of the foot. If preoperative imaging showed intact run-off to the anterior or posterior tibial arteries it should be possible to feel those pulses. If run-off is to peroneal, there should be at least a good Doppler signal over one of the foot arteries. If there is any doubt over graft function perform an 'on-table' angiogram to check from proximal anastomosis to foot.

15 Close the incisions in two layers with 2/0 Vicryl to subcutaneous tissue and 3/0 Monocryl subcuticular to skin.

Femoro-popliteal bypass below knee[*]

Indications for surgery

- Ischaemia due to occlusive disease of the superficial femoral and popliteal arteries.
- It carries lower patency rates than above-knee bypass and so is reserved for those with short distance calf claudication or critical ischaemia.

Possible conduits

- Patency is better with vein (reversed or *in situ*).
- If no vein of a suitable size and length available from legs or arms then PTFE with or without a vein cuff (see p. 308) can be used.

Anaesthesia, preparation, and draping

As for above-knee femoro-popliteal bypass (p. 290).

Incision and exposure

- Oblique or vertical groin incision to expose and sling the CFA, SFA, and profunda artery (see p. 198).
- Medial incision below knee to expose the below-knee popliteal artery (see p. 200).

Procedure

This is similar to that for the above-knee femoro-popliteal bypass but the following should be noted.

- Consider first exposing the distal artery to determine run-off in cases of questionable feasibility.
- Take care to preserve the GSV in the exposure of the popliteal artery.
- Make sure the knee is straightened before cutting the graft to length.
- The graft may be tunnelled subcutaneously or deep to sartorius. The graft angulation in travelling from the superficial plane down to the artery is less marked than with the above-knee anastomosis and so an in situ graft also works well. However, the hamstring tendons may require division to allow a satisfactory lie for a superficially running graft.
- Use 6/0 Prolene for distal anastomosis.
- Angiography is more likely to be required at completion to confirm a satisfactory graft and run-off.

[*] OPCS codes. Elective: L59.2 (prosthetic); L59.3 (vein). Emergency: L58.2 (prosthetic), L58.3 (vein).

Femoro-distal bypass graft: introduction[*]

Indications and requirements for surgery

- Surgery is indicated when *all* of the following four criteria are met.
  - The limb is threatened (there is rest pain, gangrene, or ischaemic ulceration).
  - There is infrainguinal disease affecting the crural (calf) arteries (± SFA and popliteal artery).
  - There is good run-in (i.e. tackle aorto-iliac disease first—it may avoid the need for distal bypass).
  - There is a distal artery in the calf or foot that will provide run-off for the graft into the foot.
- Adequate vein for use as a graft is definitely preferable but PTFE can be used instead if absolutely necessary.

Options in femoro-distal bypass grafting

- Proximal level of anastomosis is usually CFA because of disease in the SFA but could be more distal (i.e. SFA or popliteal artery if arteries above look very good). An occluded SFA can be divided up to 3cm below its origin and endarterectomized to provide run-in to a vein graft if the latter isn't quite adequate to reach the CFA.
- Distal anastomosis is usually to the highest main artery in the calf or foot that will give-run off into the foot (even if it does not reach the foot itself, i.e. the peroneal artery).
- Graft material.
  - Ideally a single length of vein that can be used in situ (with valves cut and tributaries ligated) or reversed.
  - If vein graft is insufficient and the popliteal artery is open as an isolated segment consider PTFE graft between CFA and popliteal artery and then a sequential vein graft from popliteal distally.
  - If vein is insufficient and popliteal artery not open, consider composite PTFE–vein graft with PTFE segment proximally.
  - If there is almost no vein, consider PTFE graft with a vein cuff at the distal anastomosis.

Anaesthesia, preparation, and draping As for above-knee femoro-popliteal bypass graft (p. 290).

Incision and approach

- Oblique or vertical groin incision to expose CFA/proximal SFA.
- For distal vessel see Chapter 12.

---

[*] OPCS codes. Elective: femoro-tibial: L59.4 (prosthetic); L59.5 (vein). Femoro-peroneal: L59.6 (prosthetic); L59.7 (vein). Emergency: femoro-tibial: L58.4 (prosthetic); L58.5 (vein). Femoro-peroneal: L58.6 (prosthetic); L58.7 (vein).

Femoro-distal bypass graft using vein

1   Sling CFA at inguinal ligament and origins of profunda artery and SFA.

2   Expose selected distal vessel (see Chapter 12) and mobilize sufficiently to place two fine silastic slings 1.5cm apart.

3   Expose GSV in groin and distally where you would expect to divide it at graft length. Decide whether to do a reversed vein or in situ vein bypass graft. If the GSV comes from the other leg, it is usually reversed on transfer. If the vein is on the small side (it needs to be at least 4mm diameter when distended) then an in situ graft puts the smaller end of the graft on to the smaller artery and thus reduces size mismatch. Otherwise, the decision is down to surgeon preference.

Reversed vein bypass graft

4a   Mobilize the vein for the length you require, reaching it through a series of short incisions along the vein and lifting up the skin bridges as necessary to divide all the tributaries, using 3/0 silk on the graft side and the same or a Ligaclip on the other.

5a   Divide the vein at the sapheno-femoral junction and distally, leaving the graft side unsecured. Remove the vein from the leg and place in saline mixed with 30mg papaverine. Take it across to the Mayo tray or sterile trolley and, working under a good light, gently flush the graft with saline via a cannula inserted distally whilst compressing the proximal end, looking for leaks. Neglected tributaries that leak can be tied with 3/0 silk. If there is a small tear in the vein secure it with a 6/0 Prolene 'z' stitch.

6a   Create a tunnel between CFA and distal anastomosis site using a tunnelling device. If the graft is to the posterior tibial or peroneal arteries in the upper calf, this is usually a single tunnel that runs deep to sartorius muscle in the thigh and emerges deep in the calf calf incision. If the anatomosis is to the posterior tibial at the ankle or the dorsalis pedis, the tunneller is run subcutaneously and brought out at its full length in the lower medial calf and, if necessary, an extension to the tunnel created using an aortic clamp. A graft to the anterior tibial artery can run SC anterolaterally in the thigh and down to the lateral calf, usually reachable with the tunneller. Alternatively, it can be taken by tunneller to a medial incision in the region of the below-knee popliteal artery (deep to sartorius) and then run in a tunnel created with an aortic clamp through the interosseous membrane to the incision over the anterior tibial artery, a shorter route if vein is in short supply. Once the tunnel has been created heparin is given (70u/kg IV) (Fig. 14.2).

7a   Lay the reversed vein in the tunnel without twisting it. Clamp the CFA, SFA, and profunda artery. Make a longitudinal arteriotomy in the CFA approximately 1cm long. Spatulate the upper end of the graft. Use 5/0 Prolene to suture the anastomosis, starting at the heel of the graft with a parachute technique and completing it with a continuous everting suture.

8a Remove the clamps from the groin vessels and check outflow from the graft at its distal end. It should produce a jet that reaches well down the leg if the systemic BP is normal. Clamp the vein graft in the groin.

9a Place small bulldog clamps or Heifitz clips on the recipient artery either side of the proposed anastomosis site. Alternatively, wrap the silastic slings twice around the artery either side of the anastomosis site and place each under tension to occlude the artery. Make a 6–10mm longitudinal arteriotomy (depending on graft size) in the recipient artery. Flush the distal vessel to make sure that run off is good. If there is local disease an endarterectomy may be necessary. Cut the lower end of the graft to reach the distal end of the arteriotomy and spatulate it. Use 6/0 Prolene to anastomose vein to artery in an end-to-side anastomosis. Remove the proximal clamp or loosen the proximal sling and release the graft clamp in the groin so that any clot is directed proximally. After about 10sec remove the distal clamp. Feel for pulsation in the distal artery and look for change in colour in the foot.

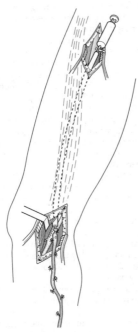

Fig. 14.2 Deep (subsartorial) tunnel for infrainguinal bypass graft.

10a Perform a completion angiogram, injecting contrast into the proximal graft with a clamp in place just above the injection site. 10–5mL 50% Niopam or equivalent should be sufficient to demonstrate the lie of the graft, the distal anastomosis, and distal run-off through a series of separate images down the leg. The alternative is to use good quality duplex scanning with a sterile probe to check the same points. Any hold-up to flow in the graft, anastomosis, or run-off needs to be dealt with at this stage to prevent early graft occlusion.

Note. If necessary two or three lengths of vein from GSV, LSV, or arm can be joined obliquely end to end with 6/0 Prolene (make sure the valves are all functioning the same way) to provide sufficient length for a reversed vein bypass graft. If using LSV it is usually easier to do this with the patient prone at the beginning of surgery and then turn them over (re-prep and drape) for the rest of the operation.

In-situ vein bypass graft

4b Expose the GSV through a series of small incisions along its length. Ligate or Ligaclip all the tributaries, leaving them in continuity. Expose the SFJ, including the common femoral vein.

5b Clamp the GSV near its top end with a small bulldog clamp or Heifitz clip. Place a small curved clamp at the SFJ to ensure maximum length of graft (to reach arteriotomy in CFA) and cut across the GSV along the top of the clamp. Use a 4/0 Prolene continuous suture, secured at one end leaving a long end in a rubbershod clamp and run backwards and forwards across the common femoral vein just below the clamp. Pull up on the suture, remove the clamp, and come back along the suture line oversewing the cut edge and finally securing by tying to the other end of suture. The cut end of the GSV forms a hood, which is usually large enough to be used in the anastomosis but if too small it can be extended by making a longitudinal incision in the graft (Fig. 14.3).

6b Give 70u/kg heparin IV.

7b Clamp the CFA at the inguinal ligament and SFA and profunda artery at their origins. Make a longitudinal arteriotomy in the CFA, making sure that the top end of the GSV will reach the length of the arteriotomy—if necessary with division of some of its tributaries in the upper thigh to mobilize it up slightly. Anastomose the end of the GSV to the arteriotomy with 4/0 Prolene in a continuous suture starting at the heel using a parachute technique (Fig. 14.4(a)). Remove all the clamps (including that on the vein) and check for haemostasis. The vein graft should become distended and pulsatile down to the first competent valve.

8b Divide the exposed GSV at its lower end, taking 2–3cm more than you expect to need to reach the distal anastomosis. Pass a valvulotome up the vein until you feel it, through the wall, reach the anastomosis in the groin. Withdraw it slightly to protect the anastomotic sutures and, if necessary depending on the device, activate the valve-cutting mechanism. Withdraw the valvulotome slowly down the graft. You will feel it catch on each set of valves which then give way as they are cut and allow the device to move on (Fig. 14.4(b)). Withdraw the valvulotome from the vein. There should be good pulsatile flow from the cut end if all the valves have been cut but often it needs 1 or 2 more gentle passes of the valvulotome to get good flow. Flow can also be compromised by run-off in a venous tributary so check along the graft again for any that you have missed.

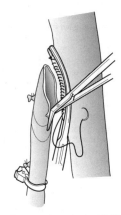

Fig. 14.3 Taking hood of common femoral vein with GSV.

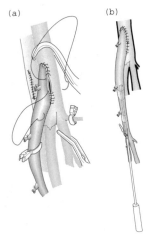

Fig. 14.4 In-situ femoro-distal vein bypass graft. (a) Proximal anastomosis; (b) lysis of valves.

9b Place a clamp on the graft in the groin (any persistent bleeding from the distal end then indicates a patent tributary). Mobilize the vein if necessary to reach the distal anastomosis site via a SC tunnel (a curved aortic clamp is useful for making the tunnel and pulling the graft through in the tips of its jaws). Clamp or double sling under tension the distal artery either side of the proposed anastomosis site. Make a longitudinal arteriotomy between 0.6 and 1cm in length depending on the arterial size. Create a hood in the vein graft by making a longitudinal incision down its wall adjacent to the artery so that the vein at the end of the venotomy reaches the proximal end of the arteriotomy in a smooth line avoiding kinking or tension with the knee extended. Spatulate the end of the vein and anastomose end to side to the artery using 6/0 continuous Prolene, starting with a parachute technique (Chapter 12) around the heel of the graft. Remove the proximal arterial clamp and the graft clamp in the groin to wash any debris away from the lower leg. After about 10sec remove the lower arterial clamp. Feel for pulsation in the bypass graft and in the distal artery.

10b Perform an on-table angiogram by injecting 10–15mL 50% Niopam or equivalent through a butterfly needle in the upper graft, below a clamp. Image the whole length of graft below this point in a series of exposures, looking for kinks or persistent valve cusps in the graft, persistent tributaries from the graft, the state of the distal anastomosis, and the run-off below this point. Mark the site of any persistent tributaries and ligate. If there is any hold-up to flow in the graft, anastomosis, or run-off it will have to be dealt with at this stage to prevent early graft occlusion.

Femoro-distal sequential bypass graft using PTFE and vein

This technique depends on part of the popliteal artery being open, either above or below knee, and sufficient vein to reach from popliteal to distal vessel (Fig. 14.5).

1 Expose and sling CFA/profunda artery and SFA in groin, patent part of popliteal artery either above or below knee via a medial approach, and the distal arterial anastomosis site.

2 Harvest available vein sufficient to reach between popliteal and distal arterial sites.

3 Create a tunnel deep to sartorius muscle from groin to knee incisions and lay in a length of 6 or 8mm PTFE (depending on distal arterial size). Create a tunnel between popliteal artery and distal anastomotic site using tunneller or curved aortic clamp, leaving the tunneller sleeve or a tape in situ to mark it.

4 Give heparin (70/kg) IV.

5 Clamp the arteries in the groin. Make a 1–1.2cm longitudinal arteriotomy in the groin (depending on graft size). Place a Roberts or similar large curved clip on the end of the PTFE graft to create a curved hood to match the arteriotomy when you cut along it on the graft side of the clip. Anastomose the PTFE to the arteriotomy with 4/0 continuous Prolene, starting in the heel of the graft. Clamp the graft just beyond the anastomosis and remove the arterial clamps. PTFE always tends to bleed from the stitch holes for a while so wrap the anastomosis up in a swab.

6 Turn your attention to the popliteal artery, which needs to be clamped either side of the proposed anastomosis, leaving at least 4cm of patent artery between the clamps to work with. Make a longitudinal arteriotomy approximately 1–1.2cm long in the upper part of exposed popliteal artery, remembering that you will need to fit in a vein anastomosis below this. You may have to do a local endarterectomy to widen the arterial lumen at least down to the next anastomosis site as the artery is often heavily diseased even if patent. Create a curved end to the PTFE graft as in step 5. Anastomose the PTFE to the arteriotomy with 5/0 continuous Prolene as above.

7 Keep the clamps in place and proceed to the second graft. Lay the reversed vein in the distal tunnel. Make a longitudinal incision in the popliteal artery below the previous arteriotomy, approximately 1cm long (depending on the size of the vein). Spatulate the proximal end of the vein and anastomose vein to artery using continuous 5/0 or 6/0 Prolene as above. Leave the clamps in place. You do not want stagnant blood in the PTFE graft, which is liable to clot. Until you complete the distal anastomosis the blood flow has little or no run-off.

8 Gently pull the vein graft down in the distal incision so that it is straight but not tight (if the middle anastomoses are in the above-knee popliteal artery remember to straighten the leg to

adjust length). Isolate a 2cm length of distal artery between double looped slings, bulldog clamps, or Heifitz clips. Make a 7–10mm arteriotomy depending on vein size. Cut the vein to length and fashion a hood. Anastomose vein to artery with 6/0 continuous Prolene.

9   Once all anastomoses are complete all the clamps can be removed so that there is continuous flow from groin to distal anastomosis. Check for haemostasis, reclamping and repairing if necessary but remembering that PTFE tends to bleed significantly from stitch holes and these should all seal up if you apply gentle local pressure and wait. Further sutures create more stitch holes to bleed! Heparin reversal with protamine may be useful to speed up haemostasis.

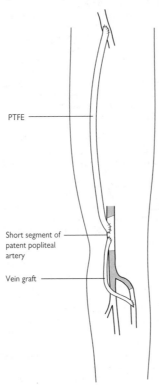

PTFE

Short segment of patent popliteal artery

Vein graft

Fig. 14.5 Sequential bypass graft with PTFE and vein.

Composite femoro-distal bypass graft using PTFE and vein

This is a compromise when there is insufficient vein for a full length graft and no isolated popliteal segment available as a relay point (Fig. 14.6).

1 Expose and sling main arteries in groin and distal patent artery. Measure the required length of graft needed to reach between the CFA and distal vessel.

2 Harvest the maximum length of usable vein (> 4mm diameter) from GSV, LSV, or arm veins (usually one piece but occasionally two—increasing the number of anastomoses within the graft makes it more susceptible to thrombosis).

3 Reverse the vein and spatulate the top end. Measure the vein against the required graft length and make up the deficiency with 6 or 8mm PTFE depending on size of vein, allowing 2–3cm surplus. Place a Roberts or other similar large curved clip across the end of the PTFE graft and cut along it to create a curved hood to match that on the vein. Anastomose vein end-to-end to PTFE using 4/0 or 5/0 Prolene.

4 Make a SC tunnel between the two skin incisions. If heading for ankle or foot arteries it may be necessary to bring the tunneller out in the upper calf and create an extension to the required end point using a curved aortic clamp.

5 Give 70u/kg heparin IV.

6 Lay the composite graft in the tunnel with PTFE at the groin end.

7 Control the distal artery between tensioned double slings, bulldog clamps, or Heifitz clips spaced approximately 2cm apart. Make a longitudinal arteriotomy, flush out the opened artery with saline, and check run-off by the ease with which saline can be infused into the distal artery using a cannula on a syringe. The arteriotomy may have to be extended distally to open up any adjacent stenosis. Spatulate the vein end of the graft to match the arteriotomy and anastomose it to the arteriotomy using 6/0 continuous Prolene. Leave the clamps/slings in place while you turn your attention to the top end of the graft.

8 Clamp the groin arteries and make a longitudinal arteriotomy in the CFA approximately 1–1.2cm long (depending on size of PTFE used). Straighten the leg and pull the composite graft up in the groin so that it is straight but not tight. Cut the PTFE to length so that it reaches a millimetre or so beyond the top end of the arteriotomy. Spatulate the end of the PTFE to match the arteriotomy using a curved clip as above. Anastomose graft to artery using 4/0 continuous Prolene. Remove the proximal clamp/sling on the distal artery and the groin clamps so that any debris is diverted away from the distal leg. After about 10sec remove the distal sling/clamp.

9 Check for pulsation in the distal graft and artery and look for improved colour in the foot. Check for haemostasis, reclamping and repairing as necessary, but remembering that PTFE will bleed from stitch holes for some time and making new stitch holes does not

help. Gentle pressure from a gauze swab plus protamine to reverse the heparin, if necessary, will help.

10 Perform an on-table angiogram with a butterfly needle in the PTFE graft in the groin and a clamp above this point. Use 10–15mL 50% Niopam or equivalent and check the length of the graft for kinking, compression, or anastomotic narrowing, the distal anastomosis, and the run-off. Correct any impedance to flow at this point—otherwise the graft is likely to thrombose soon after surgery.

11 Close the incisions with 2/0 Vicryl and a 3/0 subcuticular absorbable suture.

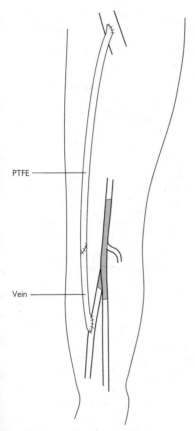

Fig. 14.6 Composite femoro-distal bypass graft using PTFE and vein.

Femoro-distal bypass graft using PTFE and a vein cuff

1 Expose and sling arteries in groin. Expose and sling artery either side of proposed distal anastomosis. Harvest 3cm vein at least 5mm in diameter from groin or wherever available and save in saline with 30mg papaverine added.

2 Create a tunnel deep to sartorius muscle in the thigh and staying deep down to the distal exposure if in medial calf, subcutaneous if in the lower leg. Lay in it a length of 6mm reinforced PTFE.

3 Make a longitudinal arteriotomy in the CFA. Create a curved hood to the PTFE and anastomose the two together using 2/0 or 3/0 continuous Prolene. Clamp the PTFE just below the anastomosis and remove the arterial clamps. Wrap a gauze swab around the suture line to promote haemostasis.

4 Now turn your attention to the lower incision. Clamp or double sling the artery and make an 8–10mm longitudinal arteriotomy. Take the length of vein and divide it longitudinally to open it out. Start at the proximal end of the arteriotomy with a double-ended 6/0 Prolene suture and secure the middle of the longest edge of the vein to this part with parachute stitches. Continue the suture line along the arteriotomy on one side until you reach the end. Cut the vein across at this point and continue round on to the other side of the arteriotomy, now stitching to the shorter side of the vein until you reach the next corner on the vein patch. Tie the suture to itself on the external surface at this point. Take the other end of the suture and sew the rest of the long side along the remaining edge of arteriotomy and then spiral up on to the top of the vein strip already attached until you reach the midline; then tie the suture to itself with an external knot. Cut off the redundant vein strip so that there is a flat top to the vein cuff (Fig. 14.7).

5 Cut the end of the PTFE graft obliquely to match the top of the vein cuff, ensuring that the graft is the correct length with the knee extended. Anastomose the PTFE to cuff with 5/0 or 6/0 Prolene.

6 Remove the proximal clamp on the distal artery and then the clamp on the graft. After 10–15sec remove the distal clamp. Feel for distal pulsation and check foot colour.

7 Perform an on-table angiogram via a needle puncture of the PTFE graft in the groin and injecting 10–15mL 50% Niopam or equivalent. Follow the graft down the leg, check the distal anastomosis and run-off. Place a 3/0 Prolene 'z' stitch around the needle before removing it so the haemostasis can be rapidly achieved by tying the suture once the needle is removed. Make any corrections necessary to improve flow at this stage.

8 Close the wounds with Vicryl and subcuticular 3/0 absorbable suture.

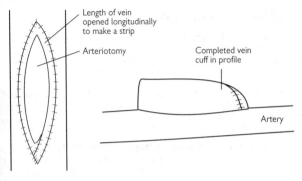

Length of vein
opened longitudinally
to make a strip

Arteriotomy

Completed vein
cuff in profile

Artery

Fig. 14.7 Vein cuff for femoro-distal bypass graft.

Popliteal aneurysm

- Aneurysm of the popliteal artery is the most common peripheral aneurysm.
- Unlike aortic aneurysm its major complication is acute limb ischaemia secondary to thrombotic occlusion of the aneurysm or emboli to the distal arteries.
- May be diagnosed after presentation with acute limb ischaemia or as an incidental finding, often in association with aortic aneurysm.
- 30% are associated with an aortic aneurysm and 50% are bilateral.
- 20% of patients with an aortic aneurysm have a popliteal aneurysm.

Management of asymptomatic popliteal aneurysm

- The natural history of popliteal aneurysm is not well described. It is generally considered that larger (> 3cm) and more tortuous aneurysms are predisposed to thrombose and embolize, but many aneurysms probably remain asymptomatic and undiscovered.
- The outcome for treatment of asymptomatic aneurysms is better than that for symptomatic aneurysms (usually presenting with distal ischaemia) but intervention has a failure rate and may precipitate limb ischaemia or loss. Without proper knowledge of the natural history of asymptomatic aneurysms in the population it is impossible to give definitive guidelines. Decisions to intervene may be influenced by a history of thromboembolic events, including contralateral events.

Treatment options

- Watchful waiting in the asymptomatic small aneurysm with regular duplex surveillance.
- Surgical bypass to exclude aneurysm: the aneurysm is usually confined to the popliteal artery and so can be bypassed by either a posterior or medial approach.
- Endovascular covered stent: currently not widely used because of high rate of thrombosis.
- Thrombolysis for an acute thrombotic event (popliteal occlusion or distal embolization) followed by bypass graft or stenting. Clearance of thrombotic emboli from distal arteries improves run-off and therefore the success rate of either intervention.

Complications

- Graft thrombosis, particularly if run-off poor.
- Leg oedema due to reperfusion.
- Thrombosis of contralateral aneurysm during recovery.

Outcome

Bypass grafts for asymptomatic aneurysms have a patency of 80–90% at 5y, but this falls significantly in symptomatic aneurysms.

Posterior approach for popliteal aneurysm bypass[*]

This approach offers excellent access to the popliteal artery from the adductor hiatus to its bifurcation. It also facilitates harvesting of the LSV for use as a conduit. An inlay technique is employed.

Indication
- Symptomatic or asymptomatic popliteal aneurysm that does not extend into SFA and has at least one run-off crural vessel.
- Not suitable for the patient presenting with acute critical limb ischaemia.

Preoperative work up
- Arterial imaging (duplex, TFA, or CTA) to establish extent of aneurysm and patency of run-off arteries (other popliteal artery and aorta should also be checked for aneurysmal expansion by ultrasound at some stage).
- Vein mapping, particularly the ipsilateral LSV, but, if inadequate, GSV can be used.
- Baseline FBC, U & E, and cross-match 2 units blood.
- ABPIs.

Anaesthetic, preparation, and draping
- GA with ETT for prone positioning.
- Arterial and venous lines.
- IV broad spectrum prophylactic antibiotics.
- Urinary catheter.
- Patient prone unless proximal GSV needs harvesting, which may be easier if the patient is supine initially and then turned prone to perform the bypass. The GSV from lower thigh downwards is often adequate and can be harvested in the prone position.
- Lower limb shaved and prepared from mid-thigh to ankle circumferentially and draped to expose this area with the foot in a bowel bag.

Incision Sigmoid incision over popliteal fossa (see p. 202), extended to harvest the LSV (or GSV).

Procedure
See Fig. 14.8.
1 Dissect the popliteal aneurysm away from the popliteal and LSVs, which may be closely adherent. Pay close attention to venous haemostasis.
2 Ligate collateral branches from the aneurysm, avoiding damage to the laterally positioned common peroneal nerve.
3 Sling the popliteal artery above and below the aneurysm. Measure the length of bypass graft required.
4 Harvest the vein graft; LSV is most accessible.
5 Give 70u/kg heparin IV and allow to circulate for 2min.

[*] OPCS codes: L59.2, prosthetic; L59.3, vein.

6   Clamp the artery proximally and distally and open the sac with a longitudinal arteriotomy. Scoop out any thrombus and identify any residual back-bleeding collaterals. Suture these with 3/0 Prolene.

7   Wash out any debris in the proximal and distal arteries up to the clamps. Reverse the vein and use as an inlay graft. Fashion the proximal anastamosis to the 'neck' of the aneurysm with a continuous 5/0 Prolene suture, starting posteriorly using the parachute technique. Cut the vein to length. Perform the distal anastomosis to the rim of normal artery leaving the distal sac in the same way.

8   Release the clamps and check for haemostasis.

9   Check foot perfusion and pulses.

10 Close the wound with 2/0 Vicryl and 3/0 subcuticular Monocryl.

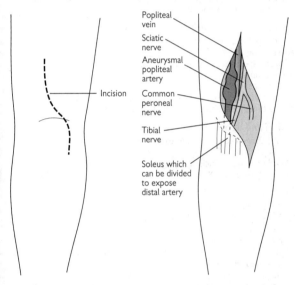

Fig. 14.8 Repair of popliteal aneurysm via posterior approach.

Medial approach for popliteal aneurysm bypass[*]

Indication Asymptomatic or symptomatic popliteal aneurysms, including those that extend into SFA and those with occluded run-off but that have actual or potential run-off arteries lower in leg. This is a more flexible approach by which any of the distal arteries can be explored and, if necessary, emboli and distal thrombus removed by embolectomy catheter or on-table thrombolysis to improve run-off. This is the best approach in patients presenting with critical ischaemia due to a popliteal aneurysm.

Preoperative work up As for posterior approach, but when the patient presents with critical ischaemia because of thrombosed popliteal aneurysm there is no time for preoperative vascular imaging. On-table angiography can be performed to check run-off.

Anaesthesia, preparation, and draping
- GA or epidural.
- Arterial and venous line.
- IV broad-spectrum prophylactic antibiotics.
- Patient supine.
- Urinary catheter.
- Limb shaved and prepared from groin to ankle circumferentially.
- Drape to expose whole limb and place foot in a bowel bag.

Incision and approach
- Medial above-knee incision to expose proximal popliteal artery (p. 200).
- Medial below-knee incision to expose distal popliteal artery and origins of crural vessels (p. 200).

Procedure
1 Dissect out the popliteal artery/SFA for 2–3cm above the aneurysm.
2 Dissect out the popliteal artery or the crural branches beyond the aneurysm.
3 In elective repair of an asymptomatic aneurysm where there is run-off below the aneurysm, the required graft length of GSV can be harvested, heparin (70u/kg) given, and the arteries clamped. When the popliteal aneurysm has thrombosed or extensive distal embolization has occurred, the distal anastomosis site (and graft length) is uncertain. In these circumstances, open the popliteal artery beyond the aneurysm and pass a no. 3 Fogaty catheter distally down each of the three crural arteries to clear as much thrombus as possible. Perform an on-table angiogram to document run-off and, if poor, consider on-table thrombolysis (5mg tPA infused over 30min) and repeat angiogram. Flush distal arteries liberally with heparin saline.

[*] OPCS codes: L59.2, prosthetic; L59.3, vein.

There may now be good run-off from the popliteal artery or a reasonable distal artery to bypass to. If no run-off is visible your options are to abandon the procedure (possibly proceding to amputation if planned ahead) or to explore the ankle vessels and pass the embolectomy catheter from here. Unless run-off in the foot can be established, revascularization is unlikely to improve the limb. If proceeding with bypass graft, isolate and sling the artery at the distal anastomosis site and give 70u/kg heparin IV (Fig. 14.9).

4   Harvest the GSV to the required length, reverse, and tunnel deeply from the upper incision to the distal anastomosis site.
5   Ligate the popliteal artery above the aneurysm with 0 Prolene.
6   Anastomose the graft end-to-side to the artery above the ligature with 5/0 Prolene.
7   Ligate the popliteal artery below the aneurysm. Anastomose the vein end to side to the selected distal artery with 5/0 or 6/0 Prolene.
8   Release clamps and check haemostasis.
9   Check perfusion of foot.
10 The acutely ischaemic leg may need fasciotomies (see p. 322).

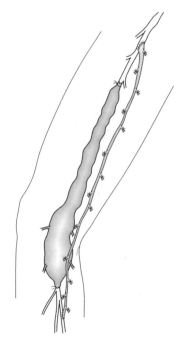

Fig. 14.9 Medial approach to popliteal aneurysm.

Femoral embolectomy*

Indication

For the treatment of acute leg ischaemia associated with embolic occlusion of the iliac, femoral, or popliteal vessels. Acute aortic occlusion due to saddle embolus (lodged astride the aortic bifurcation) can be treated with bilateral femoral embolectomies.

Clinical presentation

- Presentation is classically with one or more or the six Ps (see box).
- Acute ischaemia may also present as new onset of short distance claudication.
- Ischaemic symptoms may abate with natural thrombolysis of an embolus.
- Delayed presentation can make embolectomy difficult and potentially hazardous to vessels with adherent clot.
- Acute limb ischaemia may be part of a systemic pathology in severe illness such as carcinomatosis.
- It is important to differentiate acute thromboembolic disease from deteriorating chronic atherosclerotic disease.

The six Ps of acute limb ischaemia

- Pain
- Paraesthesia
- Paralysis
- Perishing with cold
- Pale
- Pulseless

The seventh P

- Palpitations of cardiac arrhythmia

Differential diagnosis of acute lower limb ischaemia

- Arterial embolus.
- Thrombosis on pre-existing atheroma.
- Thrombosis of popliteal aneurysm.
- Aortic or iliac dissection.
- Traumatic disruption of arteries.

Clinical assessment

- Determine duration of symptoms.
- What is the degree of ischaemia? Is there sensory or motor impairment?
- Determine limb viability—is there fixed mottling?
- Is there a past history of claudication?

* OPCS code L62.2.

- Are there risk factors for atherosclerosis?
- Are all pulses palpable on the contralateral side?
- Is there gross limb swelling with blue/purple discolouration as in phlegmasia caerulea dolens?
- Is there a popliteal aneurysm palpable in either leg?
- Is the patient in atrial fibrillation?
- Is there evidence of thromboembolism to other sites?
- Determine the position of the thromboembolic occlusion by palpating pulses.
- Consider imaging with duplex or angiography if limb not critically ischaemic and some doubt regarding cause of ischaemia.

Alternative treatments

- Popliteal embolectomy.
- Angiography with thrombolysis.
- Delayed angioplasty (after 6 weeks).
- Primary amputation if limb beyond salvage.
- Anticoagulation and await spontaneous improvement.
- Conservative treatment with analgesia and palliative care.

Preoperative work up

- ECG. ? Atrial fibrillation or recent MI as source of embolus.
- FBC, U & E, and cross-match 2 units blood.
- Consent for possible amputation if long history (> 5 days) of severe ischaemia.
- Anticoagulate with a heparin infusion if any delay is anticipated.

Anaesthesia, preparation, and draping

- Organize theatre with X-ray compatible table, C-arm, and radiographer available.
- Broad-spectrum prophylactic antibiotics IV prophylactic antibiotics.
- LA infiltration in the groin, spinal, epidural, or GA. Many of these patients have a precarious cardiac status and are best managed without GA if possible. Epidural is not safe if heparin has been given.
- Shave the groin and prepare and drape the leg circumferentially with the foot in a bowel bag.

Incision Oblique or vertical groin incision and exposure of CFA, SFA, and profunda artery as on p. 198.

Procedure

See Fig. 14.10.
1 Control the groin arteries with silastic slings.
2 Check for pulsation in groin vessels.
3 Systemically heparinize the patient and allow 2min circulation time.
4 Separately clamp all three vessels.
5 With no. 11 blade make a transverse arteriotomy at the CFA bifurcation unless there is obvious atherosclerotic disease. The latter may necessitate bypass graft or endarterectomy rather than embolectomy, in which case a longitudinal incision is preferable.
6 Extend the arteriotomy with Potts scissors to 1/3 to 1/2 the transverse diameter.
7 Lift out visible clot with DeBakey forceps.
8 Pass a no. 4 embolectomy catheter as far as the aorta (estimate this by using calibration marks on catheter). Be careful not to dislodge thrombus into the contralateral side.
9 Inflate the balloon gently to abut the wall of the artery and pull back, retrieving thrombus and using vessel loop to pull up and prevent excessive bleeding. You should not need a lot of force to pull the balloon back; the balloon can be deflated slightly to make this easier. Excessive force with an overinflated balloon will strip the endothelium.
10 Repeat until no more thrombus is retrieved and there is good inflow.
11 Repeat for the profunda, check back-bleeding, and flush with heparin saline.
12 Repeat for the SFA, passing the catheter full length if possible.
13 Assess backflow and ease of flushing with heparinized saline.
14 If catheter has failed to pass full length distally or there is not good back-bleeding from the SFA, do an on-table angiogram. If this shows persistent distal occlusion the options are:
  • a further attempt at femoral embolectomy;
  • embolectomy via a distal artery closer to the occlusion;
  • on-table thrombolysis (5mg tPA infused over 30min) into the SFA;
  • femoro-distal bypass graft if there is a distal vessel beyond occlusion with run-off to foot.
15 Close arteriotomy with 4/0 Prolene and remove clamps (SFA clamp last). Check foot perfusion. If fails to improve over 5min may need to consider options listed in step 14.
16 Close wound with 2/0 Vicryl and 3/0 subcuticular Monocryl.
17 Consider prophylactic fasciotomy (p. 322).

Causes of technical failure

• Unable to pass catheter due to adherent organized thrombus or atherosclerosis.
• Recurrence of thrombus (especially if patient has prothrombotic state or heparin-induced thrombocytopenia).
• Dissection from passage of embolectomy catheter.
• Stenosis or flap at arteriotomy closure.

Early postoperative complications

- Bleeding.
- Compartment syndrome.
- Renal failure.
- Sudden death due to cardiac arrhythmia.
- Recurrent limb ischaemia due to thrombosis (usually linked to one of the problems listed above not recognized at the end of surgery).

Postoperative management

- Keep systemically anticoagulated by beginning a heparin infusion 2h following the bolus.
- Monitor anticoagulation with 4-hourly APTT (keep twice normal).
- Monitor for compartment syndrome.
- Monitor urine output
- Plan investigations to determine source of thromboembolus:
  - transthoracic echocardiogram;
  - trans-oesophageal echocardiogram;
  - imaging of the aorto-iliac segment.
- Commence long-term anticoagulation with warfarin.

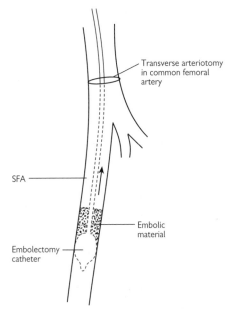

Fig. 14.10 Femoral embolectomy.

Popliteal embolectomy[*]

As for femoral embolectomy but via a medial approach to the infrap-opliteal artery, exposing the origins of the crural arteries and sweeping each of these with the embolectomy catheter via a transverse incision in the lower popliteal artery (Fig. 14.11). Used when popliteal pulse palpable but more distal embolic occlusion or if embolectomy via femoral artery fails.

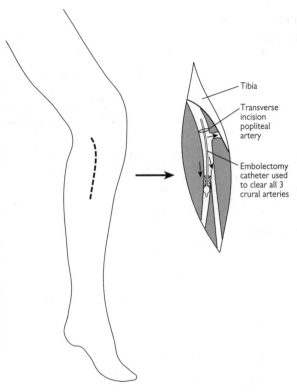

Fig. 14.11 Popliteal embolectomy.

Fasciotomy

Indication

- Fasciotomy is indicated in the treatment or prevention of compartment syndrome.
- Compartment syndrome is the clinical consequence of raised pressure within the fascial compartments containing muscle and neurovascular bundle. This most often results from muscular oedema from ischaemia-reperfusion or trauma. The syndrome comprises swelling, pain, loss of sensation, and loss of power and indicates ischaemia of the muscle and nerves in the compartment. Without prompt treatment it will result in myoneural necrosis with subsequent permanent loss of function.
- The leg is most commonly affected, particularly the anterior and lateral compartments, and, left untreated, foot drop with loss of dorsal foot sensation is the most likely consequence.
- The pressures at which compartment syndrome occurs are those sufficient to impair perfusion of nerve and muscle and are considerably less than the systolic blood pressure.

Diagnosis

- Following reperfusion compartment syndrome is likely if:
  - there has been a long period of ischaemia (> 6h);
  - there is substantial muscle bulk;
  - a high degree of ischaemia;
  - complete reperfusion.
- Diagnosis of compartment syndrome must be considered in the context of:
  - pain out of proportion to the injury/surgical insult;
  - altered distal sensation;
  - diminished power;
  - tense muscular compartments.
- Compartment pressure can be measured by inserting an 18G needle into the compartments and connecting it to a pressure transducer and monitor. Absolute pressures of greater than 30mmHg or pressure within 30mmHg of the mean arterial pressure are consistent with compartment syndrome.
- However, if compartment syndrome is clinically suspected, fasciotomies should be performed whatever the compartmental pressures.

Fasciotomy of leg[*]

Preparation and draping

- Fasciotomies are most often done at the end of a revascularization operation.
- Supine position.
- Standard preparation of the leg circumferentially from knee to ankle with iodine or chlorhexidine.
- Urinary catheter inserted (myoglobin from reperfused damaged muscle can cause renal failure).

Procedure

Four-quadrant fasciotomy is achieved through a two incision approach (Fig. 14.12).

1   The lateral incision is made over the fibula.
- The skin incision is made along the length of the fibula.
- The incision is continued through the underlying fascia opening the peroneal compartment. Care is taken to avoid the common peroneal nerve at the head of the fibula.
- The anterior compartment is anterior to the peroneal compartment and is reached either by retracting the anterior skin edge or by incising the fascia between peroneal and anterior compartments. The fascia over the anterior compartment is incised full length as with the peroneal.
- Diagnosis of compartment syndrome is confirmed by muscle bulging through the fascial incisions.

2   The posterior compartments are approached through a medial incision extending along the length of the leg.
- The superficial posterior compartment containing gastrocnemius is incised by deepening the skin incision through the underlying fascia along the length of the leg.
- The deep posterior compartment is opened by separating soleus from the tibia along its length from the popliteal vessels downwards.

3   Dead muscle should be excised. Muscle non-viability is determined by:
- dusky appearance;
- absence of bleeding;
- absence of spontaneous fasciculation;
- absence of response to nerve stimulation.

4   Muscle of questionable viability can be re-examined under anaesthesia at planned re-look within 12–24h.

[*] OPCS codes: T55.4, anterior compartment; T55.5, posterior compartment.

5   The wounds are left open on both sides and the muscle covered
    with Vaseline-impregnated gauze or similar non-adherent dressings
    and a pad. A loose 'shoelace' subcuticular Prolene suture may be
    used to facilitate later skin closure. Loose bandaging is applied.

Complications
- Failure to adequately decompress all compartments.
- Haemorrhage.
- Nerve injury—common peroneal.
- Rhabdomyolysis, acute renal failure, and arrhythmia.
- Infection of non-viable tissue.

Aftercare
- Plan re-look change of dressings under GA.
- Physiotherapy.
- Monitor renal function.
- Anticoagulation in cases of reperfusion following thromboembolism.

Wound closure
- Wounds are not closed initially.
- Delayed primary closure may be possible in 3–5 days.
- Subcuticular shoestring sutures may be gradually pulled tighter to
  approximate or close the skin edges.
- Skin grafting is required for larger defect.

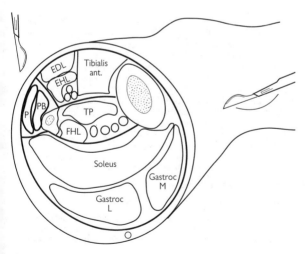

Fig. 14.12 Fasciotomy of the leg.

Fasciotomy of the thigh, forearm, and arm*

Fasciotomy is occasionally indicated in these sites. The same principles apply as to leg fasciotomy but total decompression can be achieved through one full length incision deepened through the fascia.

Release of popliteal entrapment†

Popliteal artery entrapment arises as a result of a developmental anomaly in which the artery is compressed in the popliteal fossa. The medial head of gastrocnemius is often responsible, either because of an abnormal muscle insertion or an associated band or because of an abnormal route of the artery. Occasionally it can be compressed by other muscles or bands in the popliteal fossa. It is much commoner in men.

Although present from birth it commonly gives rise to no symptoms until late teens or twenties, when it is especially found in those who have to walk or run more than normal, presumably because of the degree of gastrocnemius development. It causes calf claudication because of restricted flow and can lead to thrombosis in the artery or in a post-stenotic aneurysm and distal embolization. It is usually bilateral although symptoms are often more pronounced on one side.

Investigations

- Duplex of popliteal artery in the prone position with the foot in the neutral position and then with either active plantar flexion or passive dorsiflexion to tighten gastrocnemius. This should demonstrate a reduction in flow. Up to 50% of symptomless young men will also have a reduction of flow with this manoeuvre. It may be possible to demonstrate an abnormal course of the artery around the gastrocnemius insertion.
- Angiography should show a tortuous course to the artery at rest and compression with active plantarflexion. It may show thrombus in the artery and evidence of distal embolization.
- MR angiography will show the abnormal insertion of gastrocnemius with the consequent deviation of the artery.
- Sometimes surgical exploration is the only way of establishing the diagnosis in the face of inconclusive preoperative investigations.

Alternative treatment None.

Preoperative work up

- Imaging as above. Duplex or angiography are needed and, if there is any doubt, MRI is useful to confirm the diagnosis. This is used to make the diagnosis but also to look for arterial damage that would require local repair as well as release.

---

* OPCS codes: T55.3, thigh; T55.1, upper arm; T55.2, forearm.
† OPCS code L62.8 (division of band); L62.1 (repair of artery); L62.2 (embolectomy).

- Measure ABPIs to document any preoperative ischaemia at rest (due to popliteal thrombosis or distal embolization).
- Routine bloods, including group and save, but cross-match not needed.
- ECG and CXR unlikely to be needed in young patient unless clinically indicated.
- Decide on the basis of preoperative work up whether there is a similar problem on the other side. If this is the case then bilateral release is appropriate. In the patient with bilateral calf symptoms and inconclusive preoperative investigations, explore the popliteal fossa on the worst side with the option of making this bilateral if a compression band is found.

Anaesthesia, preparation, and draping

- GA or spinal.
- Patient prone.
- No urinary catheter required.
- IV prophylactic broad-spectrum antibiotics are optional.
- Shave and prep skin from lower thigh to ankle circumferentially.
- Drape from just above popliteal fossa to lower calf with the whole circumference of the leg exposed and the foot draped separately.

Incision and approach

Posterior approach to popliteal artery (see p. 202) with access to LSV if arterial repair needed.

Procedure

1 Identify any slips or bands of medial gastrocnemius that are abnormally attached and distorting the artery. Divide these. Check that there is no compression of the artery on passive dorsiflexion of the ankle.
2 If there is any evidence of arterial damage or intraluminal thrombus or poststenotic aneurysm formation on preoperative investigations then the artery will need opening and possibly replacing. Give 70u/kg heparin IV. Apply clamps to the artery above and below the site of constriction ± aneurysm. Open the artery longitudinally, remove thrombus, and close with patch of LSV. If the artery is severely damaged or aneurysmal then replace this segment with an interposition graft or LSV, excising the affected artery and anastomosing end-to-end. If there is evidence of distal embolization then passage of a no. 3 Fogarty catheter distally may clear embolic debris and improve distal perfusion.
3 Close wound with 2/0 Vicryl to deep fascia and 3/0 SC Monocryl.
4 Explore the other leg if indicated.

Postoperative care

- Mobilize on day 1.
- Measure ABPIs.
- Home in 24–48h.

Outcome after surgery

Almost always complete relief of symptoms in those in whom a definite compression is relieved provided there has been minimal distal embolization.

Lower limb amputations

Overview

- Patients coming to major limb amputation (around the knee) have severe leg ischaemia associated with the following:
  - unreconstructable arterial disease, i.e. too extensive to bypass; or
  - an unsalvageable lower limb because of the extent of tissue loss and damage; or
  - patient is too frail to have surgical revascularization and there is no radiological alternative.
- The risks of surgery are high, with a mortality of about 10%, because most of these patients also have extensive arterial disease of heart and brain. In the very frail it may be better to manage conservatively with dressings, analgesia, and antibiotics as necessary. Do not be persuaded to amputate just because of nursing concerns when the patient is not in distress and is unlikely to survive amputation.
- On the other hand, amputation can produce a dramatic improvement in well-being. It can convert the patient who spends their nights in a chair because of severe rest pain, who has swollen legs, who is sleepy, perhaps confused, and certainly anorexic and constipated because of opiate analgesia, who never gets beyond the sitting room or bathroom because of pain and restricted mobility, into a pain-free patient, with restored appetite for food and life whose wheelchair can take them beyond the house. The younger fitter patients may eventually manage a leg prosthesis. It is important, however, that the patient decides that the time has come for amputation. Those who are persuaded or bullied into consent will make a poor recovery.
- The other category of patients who are sometimes considered for amputation are those with a 'useless' leg (i.e. cannot be used for weight-bearing), e.g. after a previous stroke. Some have a normal lower limb blood supply but develop pressure ulceration over the heel or other pressure points and it is essential that those caring for such patients detect and treat this early with repositioning in bed and pressure-relieving devices. If conservative measures like this fail to heal a significant ulcer that is causing the patient distress, it is reasonable to consider major limb amputation. Many of these patients, however, have leg ischaemia associated with pain or tissue loss. The leg may be salvageable and the disease reconstructable but, because the leg is of little use, the temptation is to advise amputation. Always consider whether an angioplasty, with relatively low morbidity and mortality, could relieve the pain and perhaps allow healing, so avoiding amputation with its high operative mortality.
- Amputation is rarely urgent. The exception is the rare case of gas gangrene. Diabetics are most likely to get this rare complication where an ischaemic foot gets infected by anaerobic *Clostridium perfringens* which spreads rapidly up the leg, forming gas in the tissues that can be felt or seen on X-ray. It is fatal if not aborted in its early stages with emergency high above knee amputation and IV antibiotics. Other infections in the ischaemic leg can produce septicaemia but are usually brought under control with high-dose broad-spectrum IV antibiotics so that the leg can be treated by revascularization or amputation on

a semi-elective basis. Occasionally the patient fails to improve rapidly with antibiotics and urgent amputation may improve their condition if they survive it.

Alternatives to limb amputation
- Conservative management (analgesia, ulcer dressing, antibiotics if necessary).
- Sympathectomy (see p. 76).
- Prostacyclin infusion (see p. 76).

Preoperative investigations
- FBC.
- Group and save. Cross-match 2 units of blood if Hb < 10g/dL.
- Clotting screen. Correct if INR > 1.5.
- U & E, creatinine albumin (long-term poor appetite may lead to malnutrition).
- CXR.
- ECG.
- X-ray thigh if hip replacement or other metal work in situ in patient undergoing above-knee amputation to check length of stem (which is impossible to cut with a conventional saw!)

Common complications of major limb amputation
- Small areas of skin necrosis along the suture-line may be managed by local debridement of all devitalized tissue and packing of the wound. Large areas of necrosis, or exposure of bone, require revision of the amputation to a more proximal level.
- Wound infection should be treated with broad-spectrum antibiotics with more specific treatment instituted once organisms have been identified from wound swab culture.
- Phantom limb pain may be managed using analgesics directed at neuropathic pain, such amitriptyline, sodium valproate, carbamazepine, or gabapentin. Use of TENS (transcutaneous nerve stimulators) may have some benefit.
- Stump pain localized to a 'trigger point' may indicate the presence of a neuroma. This is best managed by re-exploration of the stump and excision of the neuroma.
- Depression and other psychological issues are not uncommon. They are often helped by the support of a sympathetic and understanding nurse or other close contact and usually resolve spontaneously. Occasionally specialist referral is necessary.

Morbidity/mortality rates for major limb amputation
- Perioperative 30-day mortality is at least 10%.
- 50% of vascular amputees are dead at 2 years.
- Median survival of vascular amputees is 4 years.
- Survival is significantly poorer in diabetics.

Above-knee amputation[*]

- Quickest and technically least demanding lower limb amputation, with highest rates of healing.
- Patient less likely to mobilize than with below-knee amputation.
- In those unlikely to mobilize, avoids risk of fixed flexion deformity of knee with attendant difficulties in transfer, though through-knee amputation may be more appropriate.

Alternative amputations

- Every effort should be made to retain the knee joint if it is thought possible that the patient may mobilize on a prosthesis. Mobilization is far more likely with a below-knee amputation.
- In patients who are unlikely to mobilize, a through-knee amputation will provide a longer stump than transfemoral amputation, providing a longer lever for transfer and a larger surface for balancing in the sitting position.

Both these alternatives require a good blood supply to the upper calf to heal.

Main risks

- Failure to heal—around 5% require revision of stump.
- Wound infection.
- Phantom limb pain. More likely in presence of neuroma in stump.
- Chest infection and bed sores because of poor mobility and poor nutrition.
- Only about 40% will achieve outdoor mobility at 1 year.

Anaesthesia, preparation, and draping

- GA ± epidural or spinal.
- Lumbar plexus/sciatic nerve blocks in combination if unfit for GA and unsuitable for spinal.
- Supine position (can be propped up on 2–3 pillows if awake).
- Pressure areas on the contralateral limb must be protected with gel pads to prevent pressure injury.
- IV broad-spectrum prophylactic antibiotics.
- Urinary catheter.
- Prepare the limb from groin to just below the knee circumferentially, and drape to expose the whole of the thigh with the lower leg wrapped in disposable drapes.

Procedure

The aim of the procedure is to produce a well-shaped stump of the correct length in which the bone end is covered by flaps of healthy muscle and skin without tension. This is best achieved by careful measuring and marking of the skin flaps prior to making the incision though, if in doubt, the flaps may be cut overlong and trimmed later.

[*] OPCS code X09.3.

1 Select the level of division of the femur. This should be no less than 15cm proximal to the knee joint to give room for the fitting of a prosthetic knee joint later if this is likely. Otherwise, a longer stump will allow better balance and leverage in bed and chair.

2 Measure the circumference of the leg at this level with a length of thread. Mark the centre-points of the leg medially and laterally, separated by half the circumference. Using these points to mark equal anterior and posterior flaps, with a length equal to approximately a third of the flap width (see Fig. 15.1).

3 Make skin incisions as marked above using a no. 24 blade, rotating or lifting the leg as necessary for access.

4 On the medial side, divide and ligate the long saphenous vein, if present.

5 Deepen the incisions through the deep fascia and muscle down to periosteum. Be careful not to shelve upwards as you cut through the muscle and the fibres contract; keep your blade close to the distal cut edge to maintain muscle length.

6 Elevate the myocutaneous flaps off the femur to your planned level of bone division.

7 Identify the superficial femoral vessels in the adductor canal. Divide the vessels between artery forceps and ligate them separately. Avoid inclusion of the saphenous nerve in the ligatures.

8 Identify the sciatic nerve posteriorly. Divide the nerve under tension and allow it to retract into the muscle.

9 Incise the periosteum on the femur. Using a periosteal elevator, strip the periosteum proximally to the chosen level of division of the femur.

10 Place a guard around the femur; then divide the bone angling the saw initially caudally and then cross-cutting with the saw angled cranially so as to bevel the anterior part of the cut bone surface. File the edges of the bone smooth, including the linea aspera posteriorly. If there is bleeding from the marrow cavity, pack the space with a small amount of bone wax.

11 At this point, it is useful to place the stump on an inverted receiver, covered with a towel. Carefully inspect the cut edges of the flaps, beginning with the anterior flap. Ligate any bleeding vessels evident.

12 Place a suction drain in the wound, deep to muscle, bringing it out through the skin on the outer side of the thigh. Do not suture the drain to the skin.

13 Bring the deep fascia covering the quadriceps and hamstrings together without tension and secure with interrupted sutures using a 0 or 1 absorbable suture.

14 Close the skin using a subcuticular monofilament suture, either absorbable or non-absorbable, ensuring the skin is not under tension and that there are no 'dog ears'.

15 Apply a gauze dressing to the wound.

16 Dress the stump with a wool and crepe stump bandage. This should not be too tight, as this may cause pressure injuries to the stump. Tape the drain to the bandage to prevent it being dislodged.

17   Two strips of tape stuck to the skin from about 10cm above the
     bandage and run down around the end of the stump and then back
     up to stick to the posterior thigh skin may be used to keep the
     stump bandage in place.

Postoperative care

- Suction drain is removed when < 50mL drainage in 24h, usually 24h
  later, without disturbing dressings.
- Dressings are removed and the wound inspected after 5 days.
- If non-absorbable sutures are used, these are removed after 2 weeks.
- Physiotherapy should begin 1–2 days postoperatively, with the aim of
  maintaining hip mobility and developing muscle strength and balance. If
  it is felt unlikely that the patient will mobilize on a prosthesis, further
  therapy is directed towards transfer into and mobility in a wheelchair.
  The homes of such patients will also need to be assessed for suitability
  for wheelchair access. Early involvement of the occupational therapist
  is required for this.
- In patients felt likely to mobilize on a prosthesis, mobilization on an
  early walking aid may begin at around 2 weeks, if the wound has
  healed. A graduated compression stump stocking may be fitted from
  2–3 weeks.
- Prosthesis fitting can take place at 6–8 weeks postoperatively, provided
  the wound is completely healed.

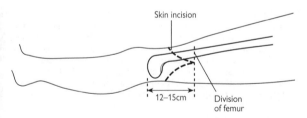

Fig. 15.1 Above-knee amputation.

Below-knee amputation*

- Technically more demanding amputation than transfemoral amputation, with significantly lower rates of healing.
- Retention of the knee joint halves the energy requirements of mobilizing on a prosthesis. Patients with transtibial amputation are twice as likely to mobilize on a prosthesis as those who have transfemoral amputation.

Alternatives The skew flap technique of below-knee amputation may be used as an alternative to the long posterior flap procedure described below. Skew flap amputation produces a more conical stump but is technically more demanding. Randomized trials have not shown any difference in healing rates for the two methods.

Main risks
- Failure to heal—more than 10% require revision of stump in some series.
- Wound infection.
- Phantom limb pain. More likely in presence of neuroma in stump.
- Chest infection and bedsores because of poor mobility and nutrition.

Anaesthesia, preparation, and draping As for above-knee amputation but prepare the leg to ankle level and cover only the foot distally, using disposable drapes.

Procedure
The aim of the procedure is to produce a well-shaped stump of the correct length in which the bone end is covered by flaps of healthy muscle and skin without tension. This is best achieved by careful measuring and marking of the skin flaps prior to making the incision though, if in doubt, the flaps may be cut overlong and trimmed later (Fig. 15.2).
1. Select the level of division of the tibia. This should be approximately 15cm distal to the knee joint to permit the fitting of a below-knee prosthesis.
2. Mark the skin over the tibial crest and measure the circumference of the leg with a length of thread at this level. Mark a point a quarter circumference round either side from the tibial crest. Mark a slightly convex line joining these two points anteriorly. This describes the incision for the anterior skin flap (see Fig 15.2).
3. Mark a long posterior flap from these points. The flap should initially extend to the limit of healthy skin distally but can be trimmed later.
4. Make skin incisions along the marks made and deepen through the deep fascia anteriorly. Incise the periosteum on the tibia at the same level to mark the level of division.
5. Divide the muscles of the anterior and lateral compartments down to the fibula. Divide and ligate the anterior tibial vessels. Divide the fibula 2.5cm proximal to the level of division of the tibia, with a lateral bevel.

---

* OPCS code X09.5.

6   Deepen the incision for the posterior flap through the deep fascia and muscle down to tibia. Divide and ligate the posterior tibial and peroneal vessels. Fillet the tibia off the posterior flap.

7   Place a guard around the tibia then divide the bone. Begin by making an oblique cut in the tibia anteriorly; then make a second cut square to the bone. In this way, an anterior bevel is created. File the edges of the bone smooth. If there is bleeding from the marrow cavity, pack the space with a small amount of bone wax.

8   Thin out the posterior flap by filleting the soleus muscle off the gastrocnemius muscle and excising it. The lateral and medial edges of the gastrocnemius muscle may also be excised if bulky.

9   Fold the posterior flap anteriorly to meet the anterior wound edge and excise any excess tissue. Ensure that both deep fascia and skin can be apposed without any tension.

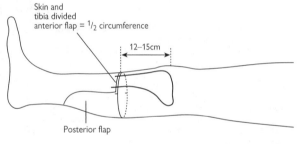

Fig. 15.2 Below-knee amputation.

10 At this point, it is useful to place the stump on an inverted receiver, covered with a towel.

11 Carefully inspect the cut edges of the flaps, beginning with the anterior flap. Ligate or diathermize any bleeding vessels evident.

12 Place a suction drain deep to the muscle in the wound bringing it out through the skin on the outer side of the calf. Do not suture the drain to the skin.

13 Suture the deep fascia of the posterior flap to that of the anterior flap and to the periosteum of the tibia with 0 Vicryl.

14 Close the skin using a subcuticular Monocryl or similar suture, ensuring the skin is not under tension and that there are no 'dog ears'.

15 Apply a gauze dressing to the wound.

16 Dress the stump with a wool and crepe stump bandage. This should not be too tight, as this may cause pressure injuries to the stump. Tape the drain to the bandage to prevent it being dislodged.

Postoperative care

- Suction drain is removed when < 50mL drainage in 24h, usually 24h later, without disturbing dressings.
- Dressings are removed and the wound inspected after 5 days.
- If non-absorbable skin sutures are used, these are removed after 2 weeks.
- Physiotherapy should begin 1–2 days postoperatively, with the aim of maintaining mobility of the knee and hip joints and developing muscle strength. Failure to maintain mobility of these joints may result in fixed flexion deformities that can jeopardize future mobilization on a prosthesis. Check daily to make sure that the knee joint can be fully extended.
- Mobilization on an early walking aid may begin at around 2 weeks, if the wound has healed. A graduated compression stump stocking may be fitted from 2–3 weeks.
- Prosthesis fitting can take place at 6–8 weeks postoperatively, provided the wound is completely healed.

Through-knee amputation[*]

- Suitable for patients in whom below-knee amputation would be technically feasible, but who would be unlikely to mobilize on a prosthesis.
- A through-knee amputation (TKA) provides a longer lever with better muscle balance than above-knee amputation, aiding independent transfer.
- A TKA also allows an end-bearing prosthesis to be worn, avoiding the straps and ischial weight-bearing complications of an above-knee prosthesis.
- TKA is potentially a very rapid and bloodless operation.

Alternatives

- Above-knee amputation has a better healing rate than TKA. It should be considered in patients in whom it is particularly desirable to avoid re-operation because of severe co-morbidities.
- In patients unlikely even to transfer independently, above-knee amputation is also the operation of choice.
- TKA requires long skin flaps so, if there is any concern about the vascularity of the skin in this area, again consider above-knee amputation.

Main risks

- Failure to heal. Healing is achieved in around 80% of cases.
- Wound infection.
- Phantom limb pain. More likely in presence of neuroma in stump.
- Chest infection and bed sores because of poor mobility and nutrition.

Anaesthesia, preparation, and draping As for below-knee amputation.

Procedure

1   Mark the skin over the tibial tuberosity and measure the circumference of the leg at this point with a ligature.
2   A skin incision is made forming equal lateral and medial flaps (using the ligature to determine half circumference) based on the tibial tuberosity anteriorly and the popliteal skin crease posteriorly. The flap length at apex is approximately 1/3 of the measured circumference (Fig. 15.3).
3   The skin flaps are reflected and the patella tendon and GSV exposed. The vein is ligated and divided, avoiding ligation of the saphenous nerve. The patellar tendon is divided at its insertion into the tibial tuberosity.
4   The anterior knee joint capsule is divided transversely to expose the femoral condyles. Further flexion opens the knee joint to expose the cruciate ligaments.
5   The tendons of the hamstrings and biceps femoris and the medial and lateral knee ligaments are divided.

[*] OPCS code X09.4.

6 The cruciate ligaments are divided, leaving them as long as possible.
7 Division of the knee capsule is completed, exposing the popliteal vessels and sciatic nerve.
8 The popliteal vessels are divided and double-ligated individually. The sciatic nerve is divided under tension and allowed to retract.
9 The medial and lateral heads of gastrocnemius are divide to complete the amputation.
10 Haemostasis is secured by diathermy or ligation of any bleeding vessels.
11 Hamstrings and biceps femoris tendons are secured to the cruciate ligaments with 0 or 1 absorbable braided suture. The patellar tendon is also secured to the cruciate ligaments, lying in the intercondylar notch.
12 After securing haemostasis, the skin flaps are closed with a subcuticular monofilament suture over a suction drain, ensuring there is no tension. The drain is not sutured to the skin.
13 A gauze dressing is applied to the wound.
14 The stump is dressed with a wool and crepe stump bandage. This should not be too tight, as this may cause pressure injuries to the stump. The drain is taped to the bandage to prevent it being dislodged.

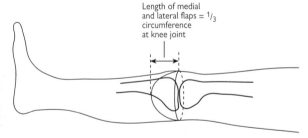

Length of medial and lateral flaps = 1/3 circumference at knee joint

Fig. 15.3 Through-knee amputation.

Postoperative care
- Suction drain is removed when < 50mL drainage in 24h, usually 24h later, without disturbing dressings.
- Dressings are removed and the wound inspected after 5 days.
- If non-absorbable sutures are used, these are removed after 2 weeks.
- Physiotherapy should begin 1–2 days postoperatively, with the aim of maintaining mobility of hip joint and developing muscle strength. Failure to maintain mobility of the hip joint may result in fixed flexion deformities that can jeopardize future mobilization on a prosthesis.
- Mobilization on an early walking aid may begin at around 2 weeks, if the wound has healed. A graduated compression stump stocking may be fitted from 2–3 weeks.
- Prosthesis fitting can take place at 6–8 weeks postoperatively, provided the wound is completely healed.

Transmetatarsal amputation[*]

Indications for surgery Indicated in tissue loss, severe infection, or gangrene affecting multiple toes, but with preservation of the web spaces. The skin of the dorsum up to the metatarso-phalangeal crease may be affected, but the plantar skin must be intact. There must be evidence of a good blood supply to the proximal foot (warm and pink with short capillary refill time even if pulses cannot be felt and an ABP > 0.7).

Preoperative investigations

As on p. 331 but also:
- foot X-ray to exclude osteomyelitis in the proximal metatarsals. May also demonstrate gas in the proximal soft tissues, indicating infection.
- if in doubt, a MRI scan of the foot can be used to confirm or exclude (at least more accurately than X-ray) osteomyelitis in the foot.

Alternatives

- Critical ischaemia of up to three digits may be treated by amputation of the individual toes.
- In patients in whom avoidance of the risk of further surgery is especially desirable, a more proximal amputation (usually a below-knee amputation) should be carried out, as this has a greater chance of healing.
- In patients with inadequate intact plantar skin for transmetatarsal amputation, but well-perfused skin over the proximal foot and ankle, mid-tarsal (Lisfranc or Chopart) or Symes amputations may be considered. Rarely applicable in the vascular patient.

Main risks

- Failure of wound healing.
- Wound infection.
- DVT/PE.

Anaesthesia, preparation, and draping

- GA ± spinal.
- Spinal anaesthetic.
- Ankle block.
- Patient supine or propped up on pillows.
- If consent also obtained for below-knee amputation as alternative because of doubts over viability of foot, then prepare lower limb up to lower thigh and drape to expose the leg below the knee and the foot.

Procedure See Fig. 15.4.
1   A transverse skin incision is made across the dorsum of the foot at mid-metatarsal level.
2   At the mid-point of each side of the foot, the incision is carried distally to form a plantar flap. This should be as long as possible and may incorporate the skin on the plantar aspects of the toes if healthy.

[*] OPCS code X10.4.

3 The plantar flap is reflected to the proposed level of bone division.
4 The dorsal incision is deepened through the extensor tendons
   (which are divided as proximally as possible) to the metatarsal shafts.
5 The metatarsal shafts are divided with an oscillating saw. The level of
   division should be 0.5–1cm proximal to the skin incision to allow for
   retraction of the dorsal flap.
6 The divided metatarsal bone is filleted off the plantar flap by sharp
   dissection and excised.
7 The plantar flap is thinned by the excision of flexor tendons.
8 The plantar flap is rotated dorsally so that it lies in apposition with
   the dorsal flap without tension. It may be retained there by a few
   very loose interrupted non-absorbable sutures or self-adhesive
   paper strips. Alternatively, the flap may simply be retained by the
   dressings.
9 If necessary, the wound may be closed over a small suction drain.
10 A stump dressing comprising gauze, cotton wool, and crepe bandage
   is applied without undue compression.

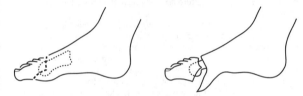

Fig. 15.4 Transmetatarsal amputation.

Postoperative care

- The drain may be removed on the first postoperative day if drainage has ceased.
- Dressings are taken down for wound inspection on the fifth postoperative day.
- The foot should be kept elevated and non-weight-bearing for 10–14 days postoperatively.
- Once satisfactory wound healing has been achieved, weight-bearing mobilization may be begun. Referral to an orthotist may be made at this point for appropriate footwear. This should incorporate a distal shoe-filler and a rocker on the sole of the shoe to allow a normal toe off gait.

Common complications

- Failure of wound healing or stump infarction requires revision of the amputation to a more proximal level.
- Wound infection is treated with broad-spectrum antibiotics until results of wound swab culture are known and therapy adjusted accordingly.
- Ulceration of the neuropathic foot may result from redistribution of weight-bearing from amputated part of foot.
- Decreased stability may result from the presence of a shorter foot in which to generate normal plantar–flexor moment at the ankle.
- Equinus deformity is a result of the unopposed action of extensor digitorum longus, extensor hallucis longus, and peroneus tertius. If severe, this can be treated by Achilles tendon lengthening procedures.

Morbidity/mortality rates Wound healing is achieved in 50–70% of cases. Mortality rate for the procedure is around 3%.

Toe amputation[*]

Indications

- Ulceration.
- Infection.
- Gangrene.
- Osteomyelitis.
- Deformity leading to difficulties with footwear or walking.
- Intractable pain.

Alternative treatment

- A toe with dry necrosis or mummification is often better left to auto-amputate rather than risk non-healing with a formal amputation.
- Ablation of three or more toes, especially if the 1st toe needs to go, is sometimes better treated with a transmetatarsal amputation.

Preoperative investigations

In order for any toe amputation to heal an adequate blood supply is required. This can be assessed by the following.

- Pulses. Palpable pedal pulses usually indicate sufficient blood supply.
- In a warm, pink foot with no delay in capillary refill, healing is likely.
- ABPI needs to be >0.7; an absolute ankle pressure greater than 100mmHg is an alternative guide. Rigid arteries (as in many diabetics) may give falsely high pressures but the quality of the Doppler signal, particularly on leg elevation, gives a good idea of whether blood flow is good or bad.
- Toe pressure, toe pulse wave amplitude, and/or transcutaneous oxygen tension are measured in some centres.
- If there is any doubt regarding the adequacy of blood supply then arterial imaging (duplex scanning or arteriography) should be performed with a view to correcting any significant inflow problems prior to amputation. If revascularization would require extensive surgery and clinically there appears to be a chance of amputation healing with the current blood supply, then it is reasonable to proceed and keep revascularization in reserve if necessary.

Anaesthesia, preparation, and draping

- GA, spinal, or ankle block.
- IV broad-spectrum prophylactic antibiotics.
- Patient supine or propped up on pillows.
- Prep and drape around the forefoot.

Single toe amputation

1 Make a racquet-shaped incision, i.e. across the underside of the toe in the plantar crease at its base, extending up each side on to the dorsal surface, curving proximally to join in the midline, and continuing for a small distance as a linear proximal extension (Fig. 15.5).

[*] OPCS codes: X11.1, great toe; X11.2, any toe.

2   The incision is deepened to the bone. The tendons are divided
    as high as possible. The bone is divided through the
    metatarso-phalangeal joint, which lies proximal to the skin incision.
    The cartilage of the metatarsal head is removed with bone nibblers.
3   The wound is washed out with warm saline. The skin is not sutured
    unless the blood supply is excellent and the area free of infection
    and the patient not diabetic. Normally the skin flaps are left open in
    gentle apposition. A non-adherent dressing, padding, and bandaging
    are applied.

Amputation of multiple toes If the toes are non-adjacent this can
be done satisfactorily. Removing adjacent toes often results in loss of the
skin bridge between them resulting in a skin deficit that, left to heal by secondary intention, takes many months. A better option is to remove all the
minor toes and bring the planter skin up and over as in the transmetatarsal
amputation.

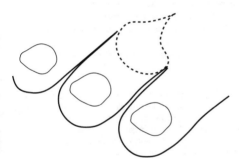

Fig. 15.5 Racquet incision for toe amputation.

Extension to remove the metatarsal head

- Indicated if the skin loss extends beyond the toe on to the foot so that there would be inadequate skin cover if the metatarsal head were kept or if there is osteomyelitis of the metatarsal head.
- The racquet incision skirts the ulcerated area and is extended proximally on the dorsum to allow the introduction of a small bone cutter to divide the distal 2–3cm of the shaft of the metatarsal. The metatarsal head is removed. Loose fragments of tendon and joint capsule are removed.

Medial ulceration of the 1st toe with preservation of good skin on the lateral aspect of the toe may be dealt with by a modified procedure.

1 The ulcer is excised down to bone. The incision is extended distally along the medial border of the big toe, splits to circle the toe nail, and rejoins in the lateral part of the tip of the toe. The incision is taken down to bone, which is then filleted out with the tendons, preserving the digital arteries as far as possible (Fig. 15.6).

2 The metatarsal head and distal metatarsal shaft are exposed and the latter divided. The toe bones are removed completely with the metatarsal head.

3 This leaves a lateral skin flap, which, if it is still well perfused, can be used to close at least part of the medial defect left by ulcer excision.

In a diabetic with ulceration of the planter surface over the metatarsal head but with a viable adjoining toe, the metatarsal head can be removed with a dorsal linear incision. This avoids further tissue loss of valuable weight-bearing planter skin, allows drainage, and the toe is preserved, although functionally useless—it just floats. An alternative is a pedicle digital artery island flap to cover the defect after ulcer excision.

Partial amputation of the first toe

Preservation of part of the first toe may be possible when not all of it is involved in ulceration or gangrene. In addition, where the indication is for toenail surgery complications, just the terminal phalanx may be removed in a procedure known as terminalization.

1 Equal anterior and posterior flaps are created at a level just below the toenail.

2 The skin incision is deepened to the bone. The tendons are cut proximally. The toe is divided through the interphalangeal joint. The proximal phalange is cut to remove the cartilage-bearing part.

3 The skin is closed with several loose sutures if the blood supply is good and there is no infection. Otherwise the flaps are approximated with the dressings, which are left in place for 48h.

Ray amputation

This is removal of a toe and its metatarsal bone. It is best suited to patients with infective or neuropathic gangrene rather than ischaemia as an excellent blood supply is required for healing. Removal of the metatarsal bone allows the foot to close together to reduce the need to fill in a large volume by secondary intention healing.

1   An incision is made around the base of the toe encompassing all dead skin and extending along the dorsal surface of the foot
2   The incision is deepened to the bone. The extensor tendons and fascia are removed. The bone is cleared, disarticulated at its base, and removed along with any necrotic tissue. The wound is irrigated with warm saline.
3   The skin is closed and the wound drained through the toe amputation site. The wound is dressed.

Postoperative care after toe amputation The patient is nursed non-weight-bearing with the foot elevated; the wound is inspected at 48h.

Complications following toe amputation

• Poor wound healing is the most common problem with toe and forefoot amputations. The risk depends on the individual circumstances but diabetes, poor vascularity, and renal failure are known to be detrimental. A balance needs to be struck between persevering with a chronic wound with limb salvage and proceeding to a more proximal amputation. Even if complete skin cover is achieved subsequent ulceration or recurrent infection can occur.
• Removing a metatarsal head redistributes the forces of weight-bearing on to the neighboring metatarsal heads, which may result in new areas of ulceration.

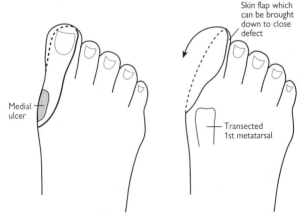

Fig. 15.6 Preserving skin flap when amputating 1st toe for medial ulceration.

Vascular surgery of head and arm

Carotid endarterectomy[*]

Endarterectomy may be performed conventionally through a longitudinal arteriotomy or by the eversion technique in which the origin of the ICA is transected.

Indications

- Carotid endarterectomy is indicated for the reduction of stroke risk in patients with symptomatic or asymptomatic carotid stenosis (1–3) of greater than 60%. It is performed as an adjunct to medical therapy with aspirin/antiplatelet agent. Patients with lower degrees of stenosis should be treated with medical treatment alone.
- In symptomatic disease, early carotid endarterectomy within 2 weeks offers the most benefit in terms of absolute risk reduction of stroke.
- Crescendo transient ischaemic attacks with significant stenosis indicate unstable disease with recurrent thromboembolic events and are considered an indication for urgent carotid endarterectomy. These patients may benefit from systemic anticoagulation with heparin whilst awaiting surgery.
- An occluded carotid artery is not amenable to surgical or radiological intervention.

Alternative treatments

- 'Medical' treatment alone with antiplatelet medication.
- Carotid stenting is being evaluated as an alternative endovascular treatment for carotid stenosis.

Diagnostic imaging

- Symptomatic patients suspected of having a carotid (middle cerebral) territory stroke should have CT or MRI brain to confirm diagnosis and/or exclude other potential causes of symptoms (e.g. brain tumour). Also useful as baseline prior to intervention for comparison in case of neurological complications of surgery.
- Duplex is now accepted as the preferred imaging technique for measuring carotid stenosis. Criteria used are:
  - demonstration of plaque at ICA origin;
  - patent distal vessel;
  - peak systolic velocity (PSV) > 200cm/sec;
  - ICA/proximal CCA PSV ratio of > 4 (quadrupling of velocity in the ICA stenosis).
- Duplex should be repeated preoperatively to exclude occlusion in the interval between initial diagnosis and admission for surgery.
- MR angiography, CT angiography, or transfemoral angiography may be required for cases of borderline patency or diagnostic uncertainty. Selective catheterization of carotid artery for contrast injection on angiography carries 1% stroke rate. Therefore it is used only when essential to demonstrate lesion clearly.

---

[*] OPCS codes: L29.4, + patch; L29.5, no patch.

Preparation for surgery

- Dual antiplatelet therapy should be discontinued 1 week prior to surgery to avoid difficulties with intraoperative haemostasis.
- Repeat carotid duplex preoperatively to confirm patency and mark the bifurcation.
- Obtain duplex report for display on the theatre X-ray box.

Anaesthesia, preparation, and draping

- GA or cervical regional block. Latter allows monitoring of neurological function during surgery (movement of contralateral hand and response to questions) as a measure of adequate cerebral perfusion. The anaesthetist should regularly check patient's neurological status and alert the surgeon immediately there is any deterioration. Sometimes this can be managed by raising the BP or increasing oxygen saturation but otherwise a shunt needs to be inserted unless already in place.
- Patient supine. Table 'broken' to allow flexion of the upper torso and neck extension on a head ring. Head turned to contralateral side. If under regional block, extend contralateral arm out on an arm board to allow access for neurological assessment.
- Urinary catheter not normally required.
- Broad-spectrum prophylactic antibiotics IV.
- Shave, prepare, and drape to expose side and front of neck up to midline and from clavicle to mandible and earlobe, exposing sufficient behind the earlobe to extend an incision up behind it if necessary.

Incision and approach

- Oblique or skin crease incision (see p. 208).
- If disease known to extend well up ICA then oblique incision probably better.
- Isolation of carotid arteries (p. 208).
- For eversion endarterectomy (p. 356) the internal carotid requires exposure for twice the length of the disease above the bifurcation.

Use of shunts

- Shunts are generally advocated for all patients undergoing carotid endarterectomy under GA, although some surgeons may rely on stump pressure (< 50mmHg) or other measures of cerebral perfusion to determine the need for shunting. Stump pressure is measured with a needle, connected to pressure transducer by catheter, introduced into distal CCA with subsequent clamping of ECA and CCA below needle so that, without flow, pressure reflects that generated at the top of the ICA by flow from elsewhere in the circle of Willis.
- Test need for shunt in patient having procedure under regional block by test clamp (see 'procedure' step 3, p. 356).
- Shunts are difficult to use in an eversion endarterectomy so a conventional endarterectomy is preferable if a shunt is likely to be needed.

Procedure

1 If proceeding under cervical block, the carotid sheath remains sensitive and will usually require direct injection of LA (1% lidocaine) during dissection.

2 Give heparin (70u/kg) IV allowing 2min circulation time.

3 If operating under cervical block check cerebral perfusion by monitoring neurological function (with the help of the anaesthetist) during a 2min clamp of the CCA. If neurological function is affected, remove clamp immediately.

4 During this time check that you have the following instruments immediately available for endarterectomy:

- ring tipped forceps;
- DeBakey forceps;
- no. 11 blade;
- Potts scissors;
- Watson–Cheyne elevator;
- fine suction;
- appropriately sized vascular clamps;
- if working under GA or if impaired neurological function during 2min clamp, shunt opened, checked, primed with saline if necessary (Pruitt–Inahara shunt), and arterial clip applied to distal limb. Otherwise make sure shunt readily available in theatre in case needed later
- patch available (e.g. collagen-impregnated knitted Dacron) if planning a conventional endarterectomy.

5 Apply clamps to ECA, then CCA. Leave ICA unclamped until you have back-bled it through the arteriotomy (see below) to sweep down any thrombus that would otherwise be divided by the clamp and swept up to the brain on reperfusion. Note time of clamping CCA.

Eversion endarterectomy

6a Divide ICA obliquely across at its origin to separate it completely from CCA (Fig. 16.1.)

7a Separate the plaque from the arterial wall by dissecting gently in the media for a short distance around the circumference of the ICA using a Watson–Cheyne elevator.

8a Grasp the ICA walls on either side of the vessel with DeBakey or ring tipped forceps and gently retract them back off the plaque, to which slight caudal traction is applied by an assistant using DeBakey forceps. Use the elevator to assist separation of plaque and wall where necessary (Fig. 16.2).

9a Fully retract the edges of the internal carotid to expose the plaque up to its tapered end.

10a Pull the plaque free gently.

11a Inspect the distal end for any fronds or flaps of media that may need to be peeled off with forceps or sutured down with a 7/0 tacking suture.

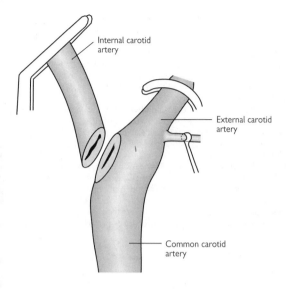

Fig. 16.1 Division of internal carotid artery at its origin in preparation for an eversion endarterectomy.

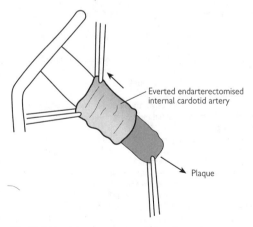

Fig. 16.2 Eversion endarterectomy of internal carotid artery.

12a Pull the internal carotid back, flush out with heparinized saline, and inspect for fronds or flaps again. Most can be peeled off but occasionally you may need to tack down with 7/0 Prolene.

13a Perform an endarterectomy of the distal common carotid to remove any prominent plaque. This can usually be done through the cut end of the artery but, if necessary, a vertical arteriotomy can be made to improve access. Loose fronds need to be removed but a proximal flap at the end of the endarterectomy, will be flattened by incoming blood and can be left. If there is no obvious limit to the proximal plaque, divide it transversely at a convenient point.

14a Flush out the CCA with heparinized saline.

15a Reanastomose the transected end of the internal carotid to the CCA using 6/0 Prolene.

16a Release the ICA clamp first to allow back-bleeding; then reclamp or occlude with forceps and remove the ECA and then the CCA clamp. After 10sec unclamp the internal carotid. Note time of ICA reperfusion.

17a Check for pulsatile flow in the distal internal carotid.

18a Systemic anticoagulation may be reversed or partially reversed using IV protamine.

19a Ensure haemostasis. Drains are not routinely used.

20a Close wound with 2/0 Vicryl to platysma and 3/0 subcuticular Monocryl suture to skin.

Conventional carotid endarterectomy

6b Make a short longitudinal arteriotomy with a no. 11 blade in the anterior wall of the distal CCA and extend up the ICA to beyond the plaque using Potts scissors (Fig. 16.3).

7b If planning to shunt put it in now, aiming to restore flow in the ICA within 4min. Place the proximal limb in the CCA and secure with balloon or clamp (according to shunt design) first; then flush through the shunt to remove any debris before placing and securing the distal limb in the ICA (Fig. 16.4).

8b Near the proximal end of the arteriotomy develop a plane of dissection circumferentially within the media to lift off the atheromatous plaque using a Watson–Cheyne elevator. Divide the plaque circumferentially at this point.

9b Lift the plaque off the wall distally until its end point where it will usually break off from the normal intima beyond. Occasionally it has to be cut at this point with Potts scissors.

10b Remove any proximal plaque in a similar fashion. There is often no proximal end and the plaque has to be divided transversely at a point in the CCA where it becomes thinner.

11b Flush the artery with heparinized saline in the direction of flow. Pick off any loose fronds with ring tipped forceps.

12b Tack down any distal flap with 1 or 2 sutures of 7/0 Prolene placed across the edge of the flap and tied externally on the artery. Flush again with heparin saline to ensure that no flaps or fronds remain.

13b Cut a Dacron patch to size, tapering at each end so that it is narrower distally than proximally.

Eversion versus conventional endarterectomy

Advantages of eversion endarterectomy

- A possible reduction in re-stenosis
- Avoids need for synthetic patch
- Reduced operation time
- May facilitate shortening of tortuous vessel

But

- It is more difficult to shunt using eversion
- Eversion offers less visualization of distal end
- Eversion may be unsuitable for disease extending cranially

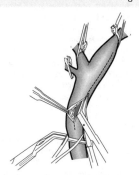

Fig. 16.3 Incision for conventional carotid endarterectomy.

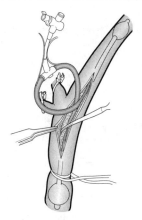

Fig. 16.4 Pruitt–Inahara shunt in place during carotid endarterectomy.

14b Suture the distal end of the patch using 6/0 Prolene on a 9mm needle and microneedle holders. Use the parachute technique to ensure accurate suture placement in this narrow artery and proceed with a continuous suture on each side until the halfway point is reached.

15b Suture the proximal end of the patch in place using 6/0 Prolene on a 13mm needle, using a similar technique and making sure that (if used) both limbs of the shunt lie to the same side of the patch. The suture line can be completed except where there is a shunt to remove. Stop suturing with a gap of about 8mm around the shunt limb and apply a rubbershod clip to the sutures with the needles still attached. Clamp the shunt, noting the time. Unsecure and remove each end of the shunt, pulling up on the slings to control arterial bleeding, allowing some bleeding to flush out debris from proximal and distal vessels, then reclamping.

16b Rapidly complete the suture line and remove the clamps, back-bleeding the ICA again first, then reclamping and restoring blood flow from CCA to ECA for 10sec before finally removing ICA clamp.

17b Check for haemostasis. Leave vacuum drain in wound if necessary.

18b Close the wound with 2/0 Vicryl to platysma and 3/0 subcuticular Monocryl.

Completion studies

- A good distal internal carotid pulse indicates a patent vessel.
- Doppler probe can be applied to confirm biphasic flow or to measure velocities.
- Intraoperative duplex can be used to detect thrombus or stenosis requiring operative revision.

Postoperative care

- Strict BP monitoring in recovery and postoperative ward aiming to keep systolic BP within a specified range (e.g. 110–170mmHg systolic) depending on preoperative pressure.
- Postoperative oxygen by face mask until following morning.
- Can eat and drink from evening of surgery.
- Continue aspirin.
- Home day 1 if support available.
- Plan follow-up duplex scan for 6 weeks

Complications of surgery

- Perioperative stroke or death (from stroke) due to:
  - distal embolization of thrombus, plaque, or strands of media;
  - cerebral hypoperfusion during clamp time;
  - hyperperfusion syndrome with cerebral oedema and intracerebral haemorrhage due to excessive blood flow in brain previously hypoperfused (usually with bilateral severe carotid disease)—uncommon.

Major stroke (limited recovery) and death rate combined is 2–3% in most large studies.

- Cranial or sympathetic nerve damage (see box) found in 20–25% patients on examination by neurologist but usually recovers and often not noticed by patient. If prolonged may need multidisciplinary management and/or reconstructive procedure.
- Bleeding should be uncommon but is more likely if surgery is completed rapidly and heparin is not reversed and if patient undergoes surgery having had both clopidogrel and aspirin in the preceding week.
- Infection is rare.

Management of perioperative stroke

- Stroke due to thrombotic occlusion of the ICA may be ameliorated by prompt operative removal of thrombus. Diagnosis by discovering loss of pulsation in distal vessel or by duplex scan while wound still open or in recovery.
- For stroke due to thromboembolism or hypoperfusion, supportive therapy with oxygen and BP control is the mainstay of management.
- Stroke due to hyperperfusion is treated with strict BP control, oxygen therapy, and possibly IV steroids.

Cranial nerves at risk during carotid endarterectomy

- The accessory nerve with high retrojugular approach
- The marginal mandibular nerve is endangered during the neck incision producing ipsilateral drooping of the corner of the mouth
- The hypoglossal nerve can be injured during exposure of the ICA as it crosses the vessel superiorly. Injury causes paralysis of the tongue muscles demonstrated by deviation to the affected side on protrusion.
- The vagus with external and superior laryngeal nerves usually lies behind (but occasionally in front of) the carotid and can be injured in dissection, causing hoarseness
- Branches of the stellate cervical ganglion in the neck can be injured in the posterior carotid sheath causing a Horner's syndrome

Disease of subclavian artery origin

- Usually atherosclerosis, which most often affects the left subclavian artery. Occasionally vasculitis.
- Often asymptomatic but can present with vertebrobasilar ischaemia, forearm claudication, or distal embolization to the fingers.
- Vertigo in association with arm exercise ('subclavian steal') is uncommon unless there is concomitant disease in other arteries feeding the circle of Willis, particularly the carotid artery.
- Examination reveals subclavian bruit, arm BP less than contralateral side, pale hand on elevation (compared to other side), and sometimes overt ischaemia of hand at rest.

Treatment alternatives

- Balloon angioplasty of subclavian occlusion or stenosis—usually first-line treatment for stenotic disease. Occlusions often too long to dilate successfully.
- Transposition of subclavian artery to carotid—one anastomosis and avoids synthetic material.
- Carotid subclavian bypass graft—can be done at same time as carotid endarterectomy.
- Axillo-axillary bypass graft (p. 422)—longer graft; requires synthetic material; cosmetically unappealing.

Preoperative work up for surgical approach

- Arterial imaging to study both subclavian and ipsilateral carotid arteries. Usually duplex gives views of proximal subclavian that are inadequate to determine extent of stenosis/occlusion. Transfemoral or CT angiography required.
- Routine bloods including group and save.
- CXR and ECG.
- Bilateral arm pressures.

Transposition of subclavian artery[*]

Indication Symptomatic proximal subclavian disease not amenable to balloon angioplasty.

Anaesthesia, preparation, and draping
- GA or cervical block.
- Patient supine.
- No urinary catheter required.
- Shave, prepare, and drape to expose side and front of neck from jaw to clavicle.

Incision and approach Supraclavicular incision (see 'Exposure of subclavian artery', p. 210). Carotid artery is exposed at medial end of this incision, deep to sternomastoid muscle.

Procedure (See Fig. 16.5.)
1. Dissect out the subclavian artery well proximal to vertebral and internal mammary arteries.
2. Dissect out the CCA at the level of the subclavian artery.
3. Give heparin (70u/kg) IV.
4. Clamp and divide the subclavian artery sufficiently proximal to the vertebral and internal mammary arteries to enable the distal vessel to reach the carotid artery. Watch out for the thoracic duct, which enters the subclavian vein anterior to the artery.
5. Oversew the proximal stump with 3/0 Prolene.
6. Clamp carotid artery proximally and measure pressure with needle in distal artery if patient under GA. If under regional block, check patient's conscious level and sensorimotor function in contralateral hand. If pressure < 50mmHg or neurological impairment remove clamp and open and check shunt (Pruitt–Inahara or Javid).
7. Clamp proximally and distally on carotid artery, make a longitudinal arteriotomy on lateral aspect of artery, and insert shunt if indicated (see above).
8. Anastomose distal transected subclavian artery end-to-side to carotid artery with 4/0 Prolene.
9. Release clamps and check for haemostasis.
10. Close wound with 2/0 Vicryl to platysma and subcuticular 3/0 PDS over a small suction drain to the deep wound.

Postoperative care
- Check arm pressures bilaterally to confirm improvement.
- Rapid mobilization and home the following day.

Complications
- Bleeding from anastomosis—should be uncommon.
- Rarely, neurological deficit due to carotid or vertebral emboli.

Outcome Usually excellent and durable.

[*] OPCS code L37.1.

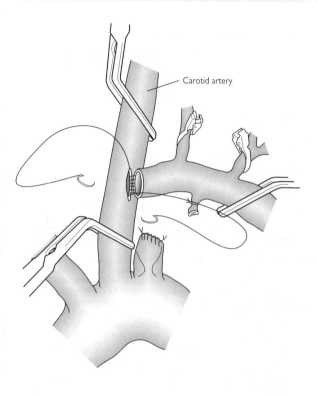

Fig. 16.5 Transposition of subclavian artery.

Carotid–subclavian bypass graft[*]

Indication Symptomatic proximal subclavian not amenable to balloon angioplasty. In a patient with ipsilateral carotid bifurcation disease it can be combined with carotid endarterectomy.

Anaesthesia, preparation, and draping

- GA.
- Patient supine.
- No urinary catheter required.
- IV broad-spectrum antibiotics.
- Shave, prepare, and drape to expose front and side of neck from jaw to clavicle.

Incision and approach

- Expose subclavian artery via supraclavicular incision (see p. 210).
- Expose carotid artery via a separate skin crease or oblique incision (p. 08) if endarterectomy of the bifurcation is needed. Otherwise expose it at the medial end of the supraclavicular incision after dividing scalenus anterior, at a level slightly higher than that of the subclavian artery.

Procedure

See Fig. 16.6.

1   If using separate incisions, make a deep tunnel between the two. If required, perform a carotid endarterectomy via a longitudinal incision with heparinization (see pp. 356–8). Close the arteriotomy using the hood of a 8mm PTFE graft. Clamp across the graft adjacent to the anastomosis before removing the carotid clamps.

2   If no carotid endarterectomy is required, give 70u/kg heparin IV. Apply clamps to the common carotid artery exposed in the incision and make a longitudinal arteriotomy on the lateral aspect of the artery. Suture the hood of an 8mm PTFE graft end-to-side to the arteriotomy with 6/0 Prolene. Clamp the graft adjacent to the anastomosis and release the carotid clamps.

3   Place two clamps on the subclavian artery and make a longitudinal arteriotomy on its superior aspect at the top of its curve, distal to the vertebral and internal mammary arteries. Spatulate the end of the PTFE graft and anastomose end-to-side to the arteriotomy with 6/0 Prolene, releasing the proximal clamp on the graft to flush out air and debris before placing the last suture with the graft reclamped. Remove the distal clamp on the subclavian artery and the graft clamp, before the proximal subclavian clamp to avoid embolic debris travelling up the vertebral artery.

4   Once haemostasis is satisfactory close the wound with 2/0 Vicryl to platysma and 3/0 SC Monocryl over a small suction drain to the deep wound.

Postoperative care

- Check arm pressures bilaterally to check for improvement.
- Rapid mobilization and home the following day.

[*] OPCS code L37.1.

Complications

- Kinking and thrombosis of graft due to excess length of graft.
- Kinking at either anastomosis because arteriotomy too long.
- Bleeding and infection occur rarely.
- Small risk of CVA from emboli in either carotid or vertebral circulation from thrombus forming during clamping.

Outcome Usually excellent and durable.

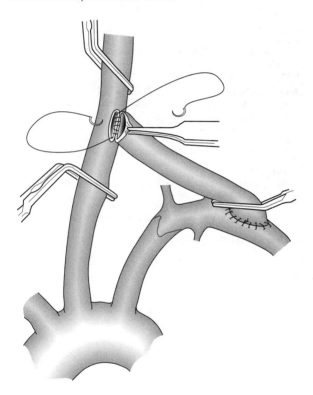

Fig. 16.6 Carotid–subclavian bypass graft.

Temporal artery biopsy*

Indication

Usually performed at the request of physicians as a diagnostic procedure in patient with symptoms suggestive of temporal (giant cell) arteritis. Ideally should be performed prior to starting steroid treatment but if necessary can be performed shortly after starting treatment.

Diagnosis of temporal arteritis is based on presence of three of the following:
- age > 50y;
- ESR > 50;
- localized tenderness or thickening of temporal artery;
- headache;
- temporal artery biopsy demonstrates arteritis with giant cells.

Anaesthesia, preparation, and draping
- Patient supine with head turned to one side.
- Select side with most prominent temporal artery. Shave temporal region and mark course of artery.
- Infiltrate with local anaesthetic (e.g. 2% lidocaine).
- Prepare the overlying skin and drape.

Procedure
- Make a skin crease incision over the artery, deepening the incision through fascia to expose the vessel.
- Isolate 3–4cm artery, clip each end, and remove the intervening length (needs to be fairly long to try and include a patch of disease that occurs in skip lesions).
- Close wound with 3/0 subcuticular Prolene.

* OPCS code L67.1.

Thoracoscopic sympathectomy*

Thoracoscopic sympathectomy is indicated for the treatment of palmar hyperhidrosis ± axillary hyperhidrosis.

Alternative treatments

- Topical aluminium hydroxide.
- Iontophoresis.
- Injection of botulinum toxin is the preferred treatment for axillary hyperhidrosis but is unsuitable for palmar injection as there are concerns over potential effects on fine motor function and practical difficulties with direct injection in this sensitive area. Thoracoscopic sympathectomy can be performed in conjunction with axillary botulinum toxin injection for patients with both axillary and palmar hyperhidrosis.

Preparation for surgery

- This is usually performed in young otherwise fit patients and little preparation is required.
- Most patients suffer from bilateral palmar hyperhidrosis. It is safer to perform separate procedures for right and left sides, avoiding the potential for potentially fatal bilateral pulmonary complications. The dominant or right hand (for handshaking) is usually performed first.

Anaesthetic, preparation, and draping

- GA. Double lumen tube is not necessary as the healthy lung collapses easily with exposure to atmospheric pressure or insufflation of a small volume of CO_2.
- Patient supine with the arm abducted and hand behind the head or out on an arm board. Prepare and drape to expose the hemithorax from anterior midline to posterior axillary line.
- Theatre equipment and instruments to include:
  - single port thoracoscope with working channel;
  - camera, VDU with White balance and anti-fog;
  - blunt 12mm port for thoracoscope;
  - laparoscopic scissors, dolphin nosed forceps, and diathermy forceps.

Incision A 2cm incision in the anterior axillary line in the 4th intercostal space (or highest space between two non-receding ribs).

Procedure

1 Separate the intercostal muscles using blunt dissection and spreading with dissecting scissors.
2 Open the pleural cavity and use a finger to confirm non-adherent lung.
3 Insert the port with the side arm open to air and advance the camera.

* OPCS code A75.2.

4 Push the lung inferiorly to allow visualization of the apex of the pleural cavity and the posterior wall. The top rib seen is the second rib.

5 Identify the glistening white fibres of the thoracic sympathetic chain running down across the ribs posteriorly and the 2nd intercostal ganglion .

6 Pick up the pleura over the chain on the second rib with dolphin nosed forceps.

7 Open the pleura by cutting and spreading scissors in a vertical plane to the sides of the chain.

8 Hook the chain forwards and divide it with scissors above the 2nd intercostal ganglion.

9 Apply bipolar diathermy to the caudal divided end. Diathermy to the cranial fibres may result in damage to the stellate ganglion with potential for developing Horner's syndrome. Twist them around the forceps and bury in the intercostal space.

10 Remove the camera as the lung is fully inflated under vision by anaesthetist squeezing on bag.

11 Close the incision with 3/0 Monocryl.

12 CXR in recovery to check for any residual pneumothorax or haemothorax.

Complications

- Intraoperative haemorrhage.
  - Bleeding from the chest wall can usually be controlled with diathermy; saline wash may facilitate identification of bleeding points.
  - Major vessel injury, which should be rare, will usually require thoracotomy for formal control.
- Pneumothorax that is symptomatic or of significant size (> two rib spaces) should be treated with aspiration or formal chest drain.
- Horner's syndrome can result from damage to the stellate ganglion through transmitted diathermy if this is used on the proximal chain.
- Compensatory hyperhidrosis of the trunk occurs particularly in patients who have had bilateral procedures and is a greater problem if the 2nd and 3rd ganglia are removed in an extended sympathectomy to denervate the axilla as well
- Intercostal neuritis is fairly common but settles within a few days with NSAIDs.

Surgery for thoracic outlet syndrome

Anatomy

The neurovascular supply of the arm comes via the root of the neck and has to pass outwards over the top of the first rib and down behind the clavicle and subclavius muscle.. The subclavian artery travels up and out of the chest, meeting the brachial plexus as it comes down and out from the spine. The two structures run laterally together between scalenus anterior and posterior, which both pass downwards from the cervical transverse processes to the first rib. Thus, both vertically and horizontally running structures surround this arterio-neural bundle. The subclavian vein sits in a more anterior plane, running anterior to scalenus anterior but still having to negotiate the space between 1st rib and clavicle/subclavius (see Fig. 16.7).

A cervical rib or band sits above the normal complement of ribs and all three components of the neurovascular supply have to stretch up over the top of it to reach or exit the upper arm. This may lead to symptomatic compression of these structures, particularly as the shoulder girdle starts to sag with the onset of middle age.

Muscle hypertrophy affecting subclavius or the scalene muscles, e.g. in swimmers who develop the butterfly stroke or in body builders, will lead to compression of the neurovascular structures.

Less commonly, a fractured clavicle that heals with distortion or an enlarged 1st rib can also cause compression.

Indications for surgery

- Evidence of brachial plexus compression (usually C8, T1 trunk) in the thoracic outlet, causing neurological disturbance, e.g. pain in medial forearm and upper arm or weakness/wasting of intrinsic muscles of the hand (supplied by T1).
- Evidence of subclavian artery compression in the thoracic outlet, causing:
  - claudication in the forearm muscles; or
  - tingling of all the fingers (especially the tips); or
  - distal embolization in the arm from post-stenotic aneurysmal dilatation of the subclavian artery;
  - Raynaud's phenomenon in the ipsilateral hand.
- Evidence of subclavian vein compression or thrombosis in the thoracic outlet, causing swelling and congestion of the arm.

Most of these symptoms are worse with the arm abducted and externally rotated because that tends to narrow the space between the clavicle and 1st rib.

Arterial symptoms are usually associated with a cervical rib or band or an abnormal bony protruberance on the 1st rib, whereas neurological and venous symptoms are often found without this association.

Preoperative investigations

- Thoracic outlet X-ray to show any cervical rib or prominent C8 transverse process that may be continued as a cervical band down to the 1st rib.
- MRI of the thoracic outlet may be useful if there is doubt regarding the diagnosis. It shows both cervical ribs and bands and may reveal distortion of the nerves or vessels.
- Nerve conduction studies are sometimes useful when there are arm symptoms or signs that do not clearly fit the picture of brachial plexus compression.
- Angiography or arterial duplex studies to show any subclavian artery compression or aneurysmal dilatation beyond the thoracic outlet. These studies must be performed with the arm abducted if they fail to show an abnormality with the arm by the side.

Alternative management of symptoms Physiotherapy to strengthen the muscles supporting the shoulder girdle often helps relieve mild symptoms. However, if there is any muscle weakness or wasting in the hand, this is an absolute indication for surgical intervention urgently. Surgery will not improve muscle power or bulk but should halt deterioration, which is otherwise inevitable at this stage.

Approaches to the thoracic outlet

There are a number of different approaches but the commonest are:
- supraclavicular;
- transaxillary.

Outcome of surgery This depends on presenting problem (vascular or neurological). There are a large number of variables in the approach taken and the cause of compression so results vary. In general, 60–70% of patients who present with neurological symptoms are improved for 10–15y.

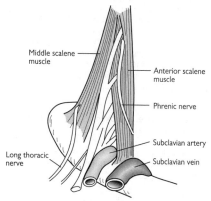

Middle scalene muscle

Anterior scalene muscle

Phrenic nerve

Long thoracic nerve

Subclavian artery

Subclavian vein

Fig. 16.7 Structures impinging on the thoracic outlet.

Supraclavicular approach to thoracic outlet[*]

Main risks

- Damage to brachial plexus or its branches. There is little room in the root of the neck and forceful retraction or inadvertent damage by dissection can cause pain (occasionally numbness) or weakness in the arm.
- Bleeding:
  - from avulsion of a subclavian artery branch—again usually due to forceful retraction;
  - from damage to the subclavian artery while dividing the overlying scalenus anterior;
  - from excessive retraction of the subclavian artery causing it to tear (it is a relatively fragile vessel).
- Pneumothorax due to breaching Sibson's fascia, which rises up in the root of the neck to reach the 1st rib posteriorly.
- Failure to relieve symptoms because of inadequate surgery. An enlarged thoracic outlet must be clearly demonstrated at the end of surgery by abducting and externally rotating the arm and checking for residual compression.

Anaesthesia, preparation, and draping

- GA with laryngeal mask or endotracheal intubation (double lumen tube not necessary).
- Prophylactic antibiotics not required.
- Patient supine, with a rolled towel placed longitudinally between shoulder blades to allow the shoulders to fall back. Initially the affected arm is out on an armboard for skin preparation and draping.
- The neck and upper chest are prepared down to 2nd intercostal space and just past the midline. Laterally the arm needs to be prepped circumferentially down to mid-forearm, a drape placed on the arm board, under the elevated arm. The forearm is then wrapped in a sterile drape and stockingette. The armboard is removed, allowing the overlying drape to fall and cover the patient's side below the arm. The arm is placed across the chest and secured here with a towel clip. It can then be moved freely during the operation to improve access and confirm widening of the thoracic outlet at completion.

Procedure

1 Make an incision 1cm above clavicle, approximately 6cm long, starting over the clavicular head of sternomastoid.
2 Deepen this through platysma.
3 Mobilize the fat pad over scalenus anterior laterally to expose the phrenic nerve lying near the medial edge of this muscle. Free up the nerve and retract medially (Fig. 16.8).

[*] OPCS code L38.8.

4   Divide scalenus anterior with sharp dissection or cutting diathermy but do this cautiously as the subclavian artery and brachial plexus lie immediately behind (Fig. 16.9).
5   Free up and sling the subclavian artery.
6   Feel below the artery for a cervical rib or band, which will tend to lift the artery cranially..
7   Clean up the rib or band down to its attachment to the first rib and divide it with bone cutters or a blade at this point.
8   Follow the rib or band up to its attachment to C8 transverse process and divide it here being careful not to leave a jagged bony end that might damage the overlying brachial plexus.

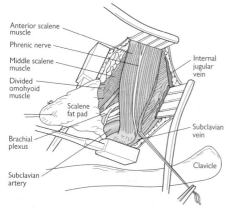

Fig. 16.8 Supraclavicular approach to right thoracic outlet and cervical rib.

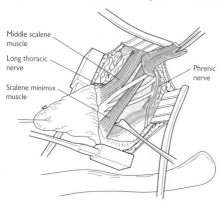

Fig. 16.9 Division of scalenus anterior via a supraclavicular approach.

9 If there is no cervical rib or band:
- division of scalenus anterior, already completed, may be sufficient to remove compression. Some surgeons resect both scalenus anterior and scalenus medius;
- a bulky subclavius muscle can be divided to relieve compression;
- the first rib can be excised—although a larger operation this is the only manoeuvre guaranteed to relieve thoracic outlet compression if there is no cervical rib or band to remove.

10 Removal of the first rib can be completed via the supraclavicular incision. It is divided at its junction with the sternum and the transverse process of T1.

11 If there is post-stenotic dilatation of the subclavian artery with intraluminal thrombus on duplex, this will need resecting and replacement with an interposition vein graft. If axillary artery access is required for this it can be exposed via an infraclavicular incision (p. 212).

12 Check haemostasis and look for a pleural leak by filling the cavity of the wound with saline and asking the anaesthetist to forcibly inflate the lungs while you look for bubbles escaping through the saline.

13 If there is an air leak then leave an underwater seal drain in the wound; otherwise a simple 'Minivac' drain will suffice.

14 Close platysma with 2/0 Vicryl and skin with a subcuticular absorbable monofilament suture (3/0 or 4/0).

Postoperative management

- CXR in recovery. Usually any pneumothorax is small and can be watched. Aspiration or (rarely) chest drain may be required.
- Analgesia—morphine in the first 24h; then regular NSAIDs for a week.
- If patient has a lot of shoulder girdle muscle spasm and pain, regular oral diazepam will help in combination with analgesia.
- Any drains can usually be removed within 1–2 days and patient discharged shortly afterwards with no specific restrictions on activities.

Transaxillary approach to thoracic outlet*

Advantages
- Good access for 1st rib resection.
- Possible to remove cervical rib.
- Cosmetically better.

Disadvantages
- Limited access to scalene muscles for resection.
- Not good for vascular reconstruction.
- Need strong assistant.

Risks
- Damage to long thoracic nerve with winging of scapula.
- Damage to 2nd intercostobrachial nerve leaving the patient with discomfort down the medial aspect of the upper arm.
- Damage to the brachial plexus.
- Lymphatic leak from damage to thoracic duct or tributary as it arches down to join the subclavian vein.

Anaesthesia, preparation, and draping
- GA.
- Patient supine but with ipsilateral shoulder raised on a rolled towel.
- Shaving , preparation, and draping of axilla, upper arm (circumferentially), upper anterior chest, and posterior chest to scapula.
- Arm wrapped in stockingette and held abducted and flexed at shoulder, with elbow bent, by assistant.

Incision Transverse along inferior border of axillary hairline between the anterior and posterior axillary folds (Fig. 16.10).

Procedure
1 Deepen incision until you reach the chest wall and then develop a plane up to the top of the axilla, next to the chest wall. The 1st rib lies at the top. The view is limited but access is improved by the assistant lifting the arm. Take care to identify and preserve the long thoracic, thoracodorsal, and 2nd intercostobrachial nerves. The last is particularly at risk from traction on the arm.
2 Clear soft tissue and axillary contents away from the 1st rib.
3 Divide scalenus anterior at its insertion anteriorly on the 1st rib, preserving the phrenic nerve, which runs on its anterior surface (Fig. 16.11). Divide scalenus medius, which is attached more laterally, being careful to preserve the long thoracic nerve, which runs down posterior to scalenus medius.
4 Clear the intercostal muscles from the inferior surface of the rib using a periosteal elevator.
5 Expose the neck of the rib posteriorly and divide it with bone cutters, taking care not to damage T1 nerve root.

* OPCS code L38.8.

6   Divide the rib anteriorly at the costochondral junction (medial to the subclavian vein) with bone cutters.

7   Use rongeurs to trim away any bone pressing on neurovascular structures. Divide any bands/cervical ribs impinging on these structures.

8   Check for haemostasis and for an air leak from the pleural cavity by instilling saline in the wound and watching for bubbles as the anaesthetist firmly expands the lungs. If there is an air leak, leave a small chest drain, brought out separate from the wound. Leave a small vacuum drain in the wound.

9   Close with 2/0 Vicryl and 3/0 subcuticular Monocryl.

Postoperative care As for supraclavicular approach.

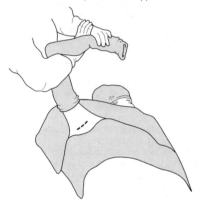

Fig 16.10 Transaxillary approach to thoracic outlet.

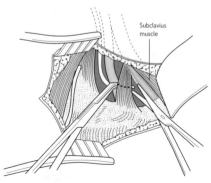

Fig 16.11 Division of scalenus anterior via transaxillary approach.

Brachial embolectomy[*]

Occlusion of the brachial artery or its branches gives rise to symptoms and signs of hand ischaemia. The diagnosis of an embolus is usually clear from the history and supporting signs and investigations. The hand has an excellent collateral circulation. Compared to the foot the presentation may not have all the classical features of acute ischaemia and it is rare that the hand or fingers are threatened by ischaemia. This allows for a brachial embolectomy to be performed as a scheduled rather than an emergency procedure in most cases. Indeed, in some cases the circulation may be sufficient that operation is not required, but the patient risks being left with hand/arm claudication or worse—Sudeck's atrophy. After about 14 days embolectomy is unlikely to be successful and the opportunity to restore the circulation to normal has been lost.

Indication Brachial artery occlusion by embolus.

Preoperative investigations

- Clinical examination.
  - Absent arm pulses. It is reassuring if there is a normal axillary pulse.
  - Capillary refill. Get the patient to lift both arms up (as in the surrender pose); ask them to clench both hands into a tight fist, then release both together. The affected side is often dramatically white or obviously slow to refill.
- Subclavian duplex—if proximal disease is thought possible, especially if the history is not suggestive of embolus.
- Venous duplex—if DVT and paradoxical embolus suspected.
- Bloods. Abnormal cell counts. Increased viscosity.
- ECG. Arrhythmia especially atrial fibrillation.
- CXR. Cervical ribs. Lung neoplasia.
- Angiography is rarely required.

Anaesthesia, preparation, and draping

- Usually under LA—patients presenting with brachial embolus are often old with many co-morbidities. Infiltrate the incision line (see below).
- If the presentation is delayed or the operation is done some time from the event, the thrombus in the distal arteries becomes increasingly adherent and removing it is painful. These patients should have adjuvant regional or general anaesthesia.
- Patient supine with pillows as necessary and arm out on an arm board.
- No antibiotics required.
- Prepare the arm circumferentially from above the elbow down just below the wrist. Drape to expose this area with the hand placed in a sterile gut bag.

Incision See p. 214.

Procedure

1   Divide the bicipital aponeurosis, revealing the brachial artery. The median nerve is medial and should be protected.

---

[*] OPCS code L38.3.

2   Follow the brachial artery to its bifurcation. A lateral branch is the
    radial recurrent artery and should not be confused with the radial. It
    can arise either from the brachial or radial artery.
3   Expose and sling the radial, ulnar, and brachial arteries. Double
    slinging the arteries is usually more convenient than using arterial
    clamps, especially if suitably small and gentle ones are not available.
4   Give heparin 70u/kg IV.
5   Make a horizontal arteriotomy in the distal brachial artery and
    remove any thrombus visible in the artery with forceps. Pass a no. 3
    Fogarty embolectomy catheter proximally to clear inflow. If inflow is
    unsatisfactory, an on-table angiogram may show a subclavian lesion
    that may be suitable for angioplasty or stenting if the facilities are
    immediately available.
6   The embolectomy catheter is then directed distally down the radial
    and ulnar arteries in turn. Retrieval of thrombus followed by
    back-bleeding and a low resistance flush with heparin saline suggest
    successful clearing of the run-off.
7   The arteriotomy is closed with 6/0 Prolene suture and the clamps
    released. The hand should pink up immediately with return of wrist
    pulses. The wound is closed with 2/0 Vicryl to the aponeurosis and
    subcuticular 3/0 Monocryl. Placing an upturned kidney dish under the
    hand to flex the elbow facilitates closing the wound.

Postoperative instructions and management

- Patients are usually heparinized whilst warfarin is introduced.
- Echocardiogram to look for the source of the embolus is rarely
  positive but should be done.

Common complications

- Bruising.
- Reocclusion—occurs occasionally. Redoing embolectomy may be
  successful—attention should be given to fully clearing the run-off. If the
  inflow was identified as dubious at the initial operation get angiogram
  to check proximal artery before proceeding.

Further reading

North American Symptomatic Carotid Endarterectomy Trial Collaborators (1991). Beneficial effect of carotid endarterectomy in symptomatic patients with high-grade carotid stenosis. *N Engl J Med* **325** (7), 445–53.

European Carotid Surgery Trialists' Collaborative Group (1991). MRC European Carotid Surgery Trial: interim results for symptomatic patients with severe (70–99%) or with mild (0–29%) carotid stenosis. *Lancet* **337** (8752), 1235–43.

Executive Committee for the Asymptomatic Carotid Atherosclerosis Study (1995). Endarterectomy for asymptomatic carotid artery stenosis. *J Am Med Assoc* **273** (18), 1421–8.

Surgical revascularization of kidneys

Overview

Indications

Surgical intervention is indicated in the following situations when balloon angioplasty ± stenting or nephrectomy are not appropriate (see 'Alternatives to surgery' below):

- hypertension due to stenosis of the renal artery or its main branches that is difficult to control with medication.
- progressive renal failure due to stenosis of the renal artery or its main branches.

Alternatives to surgery

- Percutaneous balloon angioplasty of renal artery stenosis is generally the favoured option unless:
  - the stenosis is at the renal artery origin in which case it may be possible to stent it open;
  - access to the renal artery is impossible from the groin because of occlusive disease;
  - abdominal aortic surgery is planned.
- Nephrectomy when hypertension is caused by a shrunken kidney with minimal renal function.

Preoperative investigations

- Angiogram (transfemoral or CT) to confirm site and extent of renal artery disease (duplex is usually inadequate for this) and, if necessary, to check splenic, hepatic, or iliac arteries as potential grafts or sites for proximal anastomosis. Contrast load needs to be minimized with poor renal function.
- Renal vein renin to confirm nature of hypertension and responsible kidney if this is the indication.
- Ultrasound of kidneys (not worth revascularization unless > 8cm length).
- MAG3 or DMSA scan to evaluate renal function may be helpful.
- Cardiac assessment (e.g. stress echo).
- Routine bloods (U & E, creatinine, FBC; include glucose and cholesterol if not already known).
- Cross-match 4 units blood.

Surgical options for revascularization

- Transaortic endarterectomy. Used for renal artery origin stenosis only, particularly in conjunction with aortic grafting for aneurysm or occlusive disease (renal origin stenosis is often found when extensive aortic atherosclerosis causes infrarenal aortic occlusion).
- Aorto-renal bypass graft—for origin or more distal stenosis.
- Spleno-renal, hepato-renal, or ilio-renal bypass grafting. For origin or distal stenosis when the patient has significant cardiac disease and you wish to avoid aortic clamping (spleno–left renal, hepato–right renal).
- Removal of the kidney from its bed, cooling, correction/bypass of stenoses in renal artery branches. and re-implantation (specialized surgery not described here).

All but the last approach allow the kidney to rest undisturbed in its bed so that collateral (capsular) blood supply (which is usually well developed in response to the stenosis) is preserved.

Postoperative instructions and management
- Maintain adequate filling to maintain systolic pressure between 110 and 140mmHg.
- Measure urine output hourly and, if low, increase IV fluids to push CVP up to 12–15mmHg if lower than this.
- Re-introduce antihypertensive medication cautiously as requirement will be reduced.
- Persistent drop in CVP despite adequate IV fluids, in the absence of a diuresis, should suggest intraabdominal bleeding. Check Hb and clotting urgently and consider re-exploration.
- Check creatinine daily.
- A fall in creatinine or BP implies successful revascularization. If there are doubts, duplex ultrasonography may detect renal artery flow but is sometimes too uncomfortable in the postoperative period. Alternatively, transfemoral or CT angiography will answer the question.

Management of common complications
- Graft occlusion. Consider re-exploration, graft thrombectomy (only in first 12h post-occlusion if vein), or regrafting if the patient's condition allows.
- Impaired renal function. If graft functioning this may be due to suprarenal clamp causing acute tubular necrosis. Supportive care with dialysis if necessary until recovery.
- Myocardial infarction. Systemic heparinization if stable 24h postsurgery but avoid tPA.
- Bleeding—check clotting and correct if necessary. Laparotomy at an early stage if persistent despite corrected clotting.

Results of open surgical revascularization
- Primary patency is significantly better than balloon angioplasty but overall patencies (including secondary patency rates of radiological intervention) are similar (90–95% at 2 years in some studies).
- More likely to be used in elderly atherosclerotic patients where improvement in BP is significant but modest.
- Stabilizes impaired renal function in most patients; improves it in a few.

Transaortic endarterectomy[*]

In its simplest form this consists of a transverse incision in the aorta at the level of the renal arteries to allow endarterectomy of both origins, then closure with a synthetic patch. More often it is part of more extensive aortic surgery involving an infrarenal bypass graft for aortic aneurysm or occlusive disease.

Main risks

- Further deterioration in renal function because of either renal embolization or the suprarenal clamp required for control.
- Myocardial event due to aortic clamp.
- Bleeding from arteriotomy.

Anaesthesia, preparation, and draping

- GA ± epidural.
- Patient supine.
- Broad-spectrum prophylactic antibiotics IV.
- Urinary catheter.
- Shave and prepare abdominal wall from nipples to pubis and drape to expose from xiphisternum to pubis.

Incision and approach Midline incision, transabdominal approach (p. 192).

Procedure

1 Mobilize 4th part of duodenum off aorta.
2 Clear anterior and lateral walls of aorta up to and above the left renal vein. This allows the renal arteries to be seen coming off the aorta at the level of the renal vein.
3 Free the renal vein from the anterior wall of the aorta and sling it so that it can be retracted gently upwards. It may be necessary to divide the adrenal, gonadal, and lumbar tributaries of the vein to mobilize it sufficiently. If the renal artery origins are still not exposed by retraction divide the renal vein, which can then be tied off (with risk of some renal deterioration) or reanastomosed.
4 Give mannitol (0.5g/kg) and heparin (70u/kg) IV.
5 Cross-clamp the aorta above and below the renal arteries. Surgery now needs to progress rapidly so that renal reperfusion can be re-established in < 40min.
6 Make a transverse arteriotomy in the aorta at the level of the renal artery origins. If performing an aortic graft this incision can be curved down each side of the aorta below the renal arteries to provide the site for aortic graft anastomosis. When performing an isolated endarterectomy, extend the arteriotomy into the origin of each renal artery (Fig. 17.1).
7 Use a Watson–Cheyne dissector to perform an endarterectomy of each renal artery origin. Flush the origins with heparinized saline to remove any residual debris.

[*] OPCS codes: L25.1, + aortic patch; L25.2, no patch.

8 Close the arteriotomy with a synthetic patch and 3/0 Prolene or
   proceed with aortic graft anastomosis, moving the suprarenal
   clamp down below anastomosis as soon as it is complete.
9 Check haemostasis.
10 If performing isolated endarterectomy, close peritoneum over aorta
   with 2/0 Vicryl and perform a routine closure of the anterior
   abdominal wall.

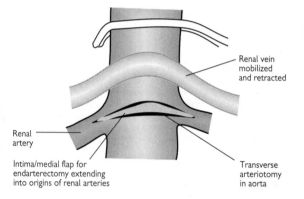

Fig. 17.1 Transaortic endarterectomy of renal artery origins.

Aorto-renal graft*

Main risks
- Graft occlusion because of kinking or thrombosis.
- Further impairment of renal function because of suprarenal clamp.
- Bleeding.
- Myocardial event because of aortic clamping.

Anaesthesia, preparation, and draping As for transaortic endarterectomy (p. 386) and groin/thigh preparation if using GSV.

Incision and approach As for transaortic endarterectomy (p. 386).

Procedure
See Fig. 17.2.
1 Expose infrarenal aorta as above (p. 386).
2 Expose renal artery for grafting beyond the stenosis (usually located by palpation of plaque). On the right this will require some retraction on the IVC—warn the anaesthetist that you may be compressing it (and impeding return to the heart).
3 Find a reasonably soft area of aortic wall, preferably below the renal arteries, for the proximal anastomosis.
4 If using saphenous vein for bypass, harvest an appropriate length from the groin
5 Give mannitol (0.5g/kg) IV and heparin (70u/kg) IV.
6 Clamp the aorta above and below the selected area or place a side-biting clamp to isolate it
7 Make a vertical incision approximately 8mm long or cut out a circular disc about 6mm in diameter at the selected point and anastomose the end of your saphenous vein graft or a length of 6mm PTFE graft.
8 Tie off the renal artery just beyond the disease (where it is compressible), control the distal artery with a bulldog or Heifitz clamp, and transect the artery beyond your ligature. Anastomose the graft end-to-end to the distal renal artery with 5/0 Prolene.
9 Remove clamps.
10 Once haemostasis is achieved, close the peritoneum over the aorta and close the abdominal wall.

* OPCS code L41.2.

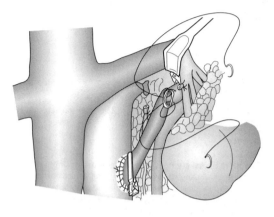

Fig. 17.2 Aorto-renal bypass graft.

Spleno-renal bypass graft for left renal artery stenosis*

Main risks
- Graft occlusion because of splenic artery stenosis.
- Bleeding.

Anaesthesia, preparation, and draping As for transaortic endarterectomy (p. 386).

Incision and approach Midline or 'roof top' curving across upper abdomen parallel to each costal margin.

Procedure
See Fig. 17.3.
1 Expose left renal artery as in aorto-renal bypass graft (p. 388).
2 Mobilize distal pancreas by dissecting along lower border and turning upwards to find the splenic artery. Mobilize the splenic artery from the left gastroepiploic artery to its terminal branches and divide it just proximal to the latter, tying the distal artery but clamping the proximal end with a bulldog or Heifitz clamp.
3 Bring the splenic artery down to the left renal artery and check for length.
4 Give mannitol and heparin (70u/kg) and unclamp the splenic artery briefly to check flow.
5 If good flow anastomose end-to-side to longitudinal arteriotomy in renal artery distal to disease or transect the renal artery and perform an end-to-end anastomosis, using 5/0 or 6/0 Prolene.
6 If splenic artery flow is poor, pass a no. 3 Fogarty balloon catheter up it gently to remove any thrombus. If there is still poor flow a Bakes dilatator may be passed up to dilate any stenoses. If flow is still poor you will have to use another method of renal revascularization, e.g. ilio-renal graft.
7 Remove clamps and, when dry, close peritoneum with 2/0 Vicryl.
8 Routine closure of abdominal wall.

---

* OPCS code L41.2.

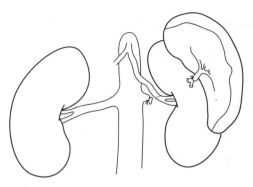

Fig. 17.3 Spleno-renal bypass graft.

Hepato-right renal bypass graft[*]

Main risks
- Graft occlusion due to kinking or disease.
- Mid-gut ischaemia.
- Bleeding.

Anaesthesia, preparation, and draping As for transaortic endarterectomy (p. 386) + groin/thigh preparation for possible GSV harvest.

Incision Midline or right subcostal.

Procedure
1 Mobilize right colon and 2nd part of duodenum to expose right renal hilum and IVC.
2 Mobilize IVC to expose right renal artery beyond stenotic disease.
3 Find the gastroduodenal artery from back of duodenum and follow it up to the hepatic artery. If it is a reasonable size, the gastroduodenal artery can be used as the bypass graft. If it is small or there are doubts about bowel perfusion in its absence (it provides a link between foregut and midgut blood supplies), then a length of GSV can be harvested from the groin for use instead.
4 Give mannitol (0.5g/kg) and heparin (70u/kg) IV.
5 Transect gastroduodenal artery to give sufficient length to reach the right renal artery or anastomose the reversed vein to the hepatic artery with 5/0 Prolene. The gastroduodenal artery can be divided at its origin and replaced by the vein graft, but if there are concerns regarding bowel perfusion use a slightly less convenient adjacent site.
6 Anastomose end of gastroduodenal artery to longitudinal incision in distal renal artery end-to-side or transect the renal artery and perform and end-to end anastomosis with 5/0 or 6/0 Prolene.
7 Remove clamps; once dry close peritoneum with 2/0 Vicryl.
8 Close abdominal wall.

---

[*] OPCS code L41.2.

Ilio-renal bypass graft[*]

Main risks
- Graft occlusion through kinking.
- Bleeding.

Anaesthesia, preparation, and draping As for transaortic endarterectomy (p. 386) + groin/thigh preparation if likely to use GSV as bypass graft.

Incision Midline.

Procedure

1 Expose diseased renal artery as in aorto-renal bypass graft. (p. 388).
2 Palpate iliac arteries and select best site for proximal anastomosis according to size, softness, and appearance on angiogram. Divide peritoneum over this iliac artery and mobilize and sling artery above and below level of anastomosis, being careful not to damage the underlying iliac vein.
3 If using vein graft, harvest appropriate length of GSV from groin.
4 Give mannitol and heparin IV (70u/kg).
5 Clamp iliac artery above and below selected site. Make a longitudinal arteriotomy approximately 8mm long. Anastomose a length of 6mm PTFE end-to-side or vein graft with 5/0 Prolene.
6 Run the graft retroperitoneally up to the renal artery.
7 Anastomose the distal end of graft to the renal artery either end-to-side to a longitudinal arteriotomy or end-to-end to the transected artery using 5/0 Prolene.
8 Remove clamps. Once dry close peritoneum with 2/0 Vicryl.
9 Close abdominal wall.

* OPCS code L41.2.

Revascularization of the gut

Overview

- Bowel ischaemia may be chronic or acute. Although the three gut arteries nominally supply the fore-, mid-, and hindgut, they link up peripherally so that occlusion of one or even two does not usually cause ischaemia (Fig. 18.1). This is particularly so when the occlusion occurs slowly, allowing collaterals to develop in size. Atherosclerotic disease, as an extension of aortic disease, usually affects the origins of these vessels. External compression of the coeliac axis by the median arcuate ligament affects the proximal artery. Tumour resection may involve proximal ligation of the artery, most commonly the inferior mesenteric artery in left colon or rectal resection. Embolic disease and vasculitis, on the other hand, can affect the proximal artery or distal branches.
- Intestinal ischaemia can present with acute or chronic symptoms and the main hurdle to proper management of either is recognition of the disease.
- The classical presentation of chronic ischaemia is with postprandial abdominal colic, diarrhoea, and weight loss but the picture is often not so clear cut and there may be a number of competing diagnoses.
- Acute mesenteric ischaemia occurs due to embolus, thrombosis on pre-existing atheroma, or mesenteric venous thrombosis and usually presents as an abdominal catastrophe with severe pain and shock.

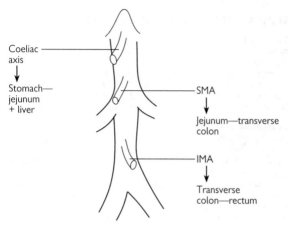

Fig. 18.1 The three arteries of the gut.

Chronic mesenteric ischaemia

- Middle-aged or elderly patient, often female.
- Presentation is with postprandial pain, anorexia, diarrhoea, and weight loss.
- Patient is cachectic, sometimes with epigastric bruit.
- Often evidence of atherosclerotic disease elsewhere.
- Revascularization of at least two mesenteric arteries is more likely to give long-term success; most single-vessel revascularizations fail.

Preoperative investigations

- Arterial imaging—usually TFA with lateral views of proximal aorta or CT angiography.
- Check and correct electrolyte disorders that may have developed with malnutrition and vomiting (e.g. dehydration, low magnesium).
- Gross malnutrition will need treatment with parenteral nutrition unless coeliac stenting is the treatment of choice. Mild malnutrition can be treated once the foregut is revascularized.
- Check creatinine; renal ischaemia is often found with extensive aortic atheromatous disease.
- Check FBC, and 'group and save' for surgical approaches.
- CXR and ECG for surgical approaches.

Postoperative management

These patients are difficult to manage because bowel revascularization leads to massive cytokine release and consequent fluid shifts, vasoconstriction, and sometimes further bowel ischaemia as a result. Multiorgan failure is not uncommon. Management needs to be in intensive care.

Bypass graft to coeliac axis or superior mesenteric artery for atherosclerotic disease[*]

Indication Acute or chronic mesenteric ischaemia with evidence of proximal mesenteric artery stenosis or occlusion due to atherosclerotic disease. Not suitable for endovascular approach.

Alternative treatment Balloon angioplasty ± stenting.

Anaesthesia, preparation, and draping

- GA.
- IV prophylactic broad-spectrum antibiotics.
- Urinary catheter.
- Patient supine.
- Shave, prepare, and drape around abdomen from xiphisternum to pubis and one groin if planning to use vein as graft.

Incision and approach Midline incision. Transabdominal approach to origins of arteries.

Procedure

1a Expose the coeliac artery by dividing the triangular ligament and mobilizing the left lobe of liver over to the right. Divide the lesser omentum to gain access to the aorta and the crus of the diaphragm between which will be seen the coeliac axis with the median arcuate ligament arching over it. Divide the ligament and crus as necessary to expose the artery (Fig. 18.2).

1b Expose the SMA by turning the greater omentum upwards, mobilizing the 4th part of duodenum off the aorta and following the aorta past the left renal vein up to the lower border of the pancreas. The SMA comes off the front of the aorta just behind the pancreas. Alternatively, reflect the greater omentum upwards, pull the small bowel to the right and find the SMA in the root of its mesentery (Fig. 18.3).

2 Follow the artery out until a soft portion is reached, usually with 2–3cm of origin. Dissect out the artery at this point and sling.

3 The origin of the bypass graft is usually taken from the aorta, either infrarenal so that the graft runs retrogradely up the front of the aorta and then curves out to the mesenteric artery or from the aorta above the coeliac axis, running the graft in an antegrade direction. It is also possible to use an iliac artery as donor vessel. The supra-coeliac aorta is less likely to be heavily diseased and calcified than the distal aorta and iliac arteries. Expose and sling the artery either side of the proposed proximal anastomosis.

4 Give heparin (70u/kg) IV.

[*] OPCS code L46.8.

5 Clamp either side of the proximal anastomosis site. On the aorta it may be possible to apply a side-biting clamp (e.g. Satinsky) to maintain flow in the artery during construction of the anastomosis. Make a longitudinal arteriotomy. Use either 6mm PTFE or reversed saphenous vein harvested from the groin as graft. Anastomose end-to-side to aorta (or iliac artery) with 3/0 Prolene. Clamp the graft adjacent to the anastomosis and release the aortic/iliac clamp.

6 Control the coeliac artery or SMA where it has been slung (double slinging rather than clamping is often sufficient) and make a longitudinal arteriotomy. If the graft is running from the lower aorta/iliac artery to the coeliac artery, tunnel it through the retroperitoneum. Anastomose the end of the graft end-to-side to the coeliac artery or SMA with 5/0 Prolene.

7 Check haemostasis. Close peritoneum over aorta with 2/0 Vicryl and close abdominal wall.

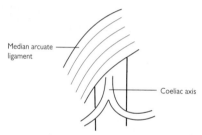

Fig. 18.2 The origin of the coeliac axis.

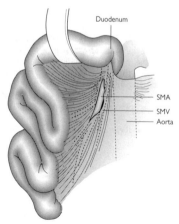

Fig. 18.3 Exposure of SMA origin.

'Open' release of coeliac axis compression[*]

- Coeliac artery compression by the median arcuate ligament is seen sometimes on arterial imaging in the context of bowel symptoms that could be interpreted as mesenteric ischaemia. There is debate as to whether such compression can really cause ischaemia, particularly when the SMA is widely open. There is often initial improvement with intervention but subsequent recurrence.
- Presentation is in middle age with epigastric pain after meals, vomiting, diarrhoea, and weight loss (partly because the patient is frightened to eat).
- The patient is cachectic with an epigastric bruit.
- Arterial imaging (duplex, transfemoral angiography, or CT angiography) shows anterior compression of the coeliac axis at its origin, possibly post-stenotic dilatation, and development of collateral circulation, particularly via the pancreatico-duodenal arteries.

Alternative options

- Stenting of coeliac artery origin.
- Laparoscopic division of median arcuate ligament.

Anaesthesia, preparation, and draping

- GA.
- Patient supine; no antibiotic prophylaxis required; no urinary catheter unless monitoring output because of dehydration or renal failure.
- Shave, prepare, and drape to expose abdomen from xiphisternum to umbilicus.

Incision and approach Midline transabdominal approach.

Procedure

1 Mobilize left lobe of liver by cutting the triangular ligament.
2 Expose the aorta at the diaphragm by making an incision in the lesser omentum. The median arcuate ligament arches across the front of the aorta and the coeliac axis emerges from its lower margin, compressed against the aorta in its proximal course by the ligament. Divide the ligament with cutting diathermy or scissors to free the coeliac axis completely (see Fig. 18.2, p. 401).
3 Check for haemostasis.
4 Routine abdominal wall closure.

[*] OPCS code L46.8.

Acute mesenteric ischaemia

Prompt diagnosis, laparotomy, gut revascularization, and resection of dead bowel is needed if the patient is to survive. Often the situation is irretrievable and the patient dies. These are usually elderly patients with significant atheroma of the coronary vessels and elsewhere; they may not survive the stress of surgery. The length of salvageable bowel may be incompatible with survival in a patient for whom long-term parenteral nutrition is probably inappropriate. Occasionally there is a history suggestive of 'acute on chronic' mesenteric ischaemia.

Causes of acute intestinal ischaemia
- Mesenteric embolus (usually to SMA)—usually elderly patient with a cardiac source of thrombus.
- Acute thrombosis on pre-existing atheroma or vasculitis. Former usually at origin of mesenteric artery; latter may occur more distally. Elderly patient who may have had pre-existing symptoms of chronic intestinal ischaemia.
- Acute mesenteric venous thrombosis—any age group, due to procoagulant disorder.

Preoperative assessment
- Classic appearance is a shocked patient with severe abdominal pain but remarkably little to find in the abdomen (at least in the early stages).
- ECG may demonstrate atrial fibrillation.
- White cell count often very high; evidence of dehydration from urea, serum amylase and lactate may be elevated; metabolic acidosis.
- Plain abdominal X-ray and CT may show some distended oedematous small bowel loops and fluid levels; gas in bowel wall or in mesenteric veins is a very late sign.
- Definitive arterial imaging is usually inappropriate because of the delay it would impose on surgery.

Treatment options
- Diagnostic laparotomy with embolectomy or bypass graft as appropriate if reasonable length of intestine salvageable. If extensive dead bowel close without further intervention.
- Endovascular approach with angiography, thrombolysis, and angioplasty as required. This has been tried with limited success in a small number of patients. The main drawback is the delay it imposes if it is unsuccessful. Thrombolysis may precipitate bleeding from ischaemic bowel where the mucosa has sloughed.

Preoperative preparation
- This is limited by the urgency of the situation. IV fluid resuscitation is essential prior to anaesthesia.
- Check electrolytes and Hb and group and save.

Recognizing cause of acute ischaemia at laparotomy

- Emboli usually lodge at points beyond the first branches of SMA so proximal jejunum and transverse colon may be spared.
- Thrombosis usually affects origin of SMA so produces ischaemia up to the ligament of Treitz and along transverse colon.
- Mesenteric venous thrombosis produces diffuse congestion of mesenteric veins in the presence of pulsation in the larger mesenteric arteries. Arterial occlusion is associated with empty veins.

Management of ischaemic intestine

- Clamp and resect any perforated/necrotic bowel prior to revascularization.
- Assess perfusion of bowel after revascularization looking for colour, sheen, and peristalsis.
- Resect any non-viable bowel.
- If remaining bowel obviously viable then perform a primary anastomosis.
- If any doubt, staple the two ends, leave inside peritoneal cavity, and plan a 'second look' laparotomy 12–36h later when any non-viable bowel will have declared itself.
- Arterial revascularization (see later) needs to avoid synthetic patches or grafts because of the potential for contamination from the bowel.
- Mesenteric venous thrombectomy is not indicated; treat venous thrombosis with bowel resection and anticoagulation.

Postoperative management

As with intervention for chronic ischaemia (p. 398), these patients are prone to major fluid shifts, further bowel ischaemia from vasoconstriction, sepsis, and multiorgan failure. They need management on intensive care if they are to stand any chance of survival.

Mesenteric embolectomy[*]

Emboli usually lodge in the SMA because of its oblique course of the front of the aorta. It is rare that embolectomy is performed early enough to save all affected bowel but it may be possible to convert what would have been extensive bowel resection (possibly incompatible with survival) to a limited resection.

Anaesthesia, preparation, and draping See p. 400.

Incision and approach

Midline incision. Check the extent of potentially salvageable bowel and determine which artery is affected from the distribution of ischaemia. If the situation is potentially retrievable (i.e. there is not extensive dead gut) then make a transabdominal approach to origin of coeliac axis or SMA as described on p. 400. The SMA is most commonly affected.

Procedure

1   Isolate the artery between double-looped slings at a convenient point 2–3cm beyond the origin.
2   Give IV heparin (70u/kg).
3   Control the artery with tension on the slings. Make a transverse arteriotomy if the artery is at least 5mm in diameter; otherwise make a longitudinal arteriotomy. Use a no. 3 Fogarty catheter to sweep the artery clear of embolic debris proximally and distally until there is good inflow and no further debris evident distally. Flush proximally and distally with 20mL heparin saline.
4   Close the arteriotomy directly with 5/0 Prolene if transverse. Otherwise use a vein patch harvested from a tributary of the GSV in the groin.
5   Release slings. Wrap the affected bowel in packs moistened with warm saline and wait 5min. Remove packs and assess bowel viability by looking at colour and sheen of serosal surface. Resect any bowel that is obviously compromised. Perform anastomosis or close ends and plan 2nd look laparotomy.
6   Close the abdomen.
7   Maintain anticoagulation postoperatively with IV heparin, aiming for an APTT twice normal. Convert to warfarin once patient stable and able to take oral medication. Echocardiogram to check for source of embolus.

[*] OPCS code L46.1.

Bypass graft for acute thrombosis of superior mesenteric artery[*]

Anaesthesia, preparation, and draping See p. 400.

Incision and approach See p. 400.

Procedure

1   If there is sufficient salvageable bowel, then explore each of the mesenteric arteries to decide on site of revascularization depending on region of bowel affected and quality of possible artery to be revascularized.
2   Proceed as on p. 400 using saphenous vein from groin in this setting where there is a high chance of graft contamination.

[*] OPCS code L45.1.

Visceral aneurysms

Splenic artery aneurysms
- Account for 60% of visceral aneurysms.
- Much commoner in women (unusual for aneurysms).
- Affect young women (often found in pregnancy) and elderly women.
- Usually asymptomatic, found incidentally on angiography, but tendency to rupture in pregnancy with high mortality rate.
- May be multiple.
- Associated with fibromuscular dysplasia, polyarteritis nodosa, portal hypertension, pancreatitis, and pregnancy.

Other visceral aneurysms
- Hepatic artery (intra- or extra-hepatic) are second commonest.
- Gastroduodenal, pancreaticoduodenal, and coeliac artery aneurysms are uncommon.
- Often asymptomatic and discovered incidentally on angiography.
- Associated with atherosclerosis, IV drug abuse, polyarteritis nodosa, pancreatitis (where adjacent).
- May rupture into retroperitoneum or peritoneal cavity, erode into the bowel and bleed, or obstruct the biliary system (where adjacent).
- May be multiple throughout the visceral circulation.

Treatment
- If under 2cm diameter probably no treatment unless pregnant or likely to become so.
- Options are:
  - ligation of artery either side of aneurysm ± reconstruction if essential;
  - endovascular embolization to obliterate aneurysm;
  - covered stent across aneurysm.

Extra-anatomic bypass grafts

Overview

- A number of bypass operations have been designed to carry blood along routes unknown to normal arteries, at least of significant size. The reasons for choosing an extra-anatomical route are:
    - the normal anatomical route is hostile, e.g. infection, previous radiotherapy, excessive scarring, or tumour;
    - the normal route would carry excessive risk to the patient because of their health.
- In general, most limb arteries are capable of increasing flow to distribute blood to a larger area than they would normally feed, unless they are significantly diseased.
- The routes chosen need to be as short as possible to reduce graft resistance but otherwise they are unfettered. They can run in subcutaneous planes and cross joints if necessary.
- Reinforced, synthetic grafts, are used most often because of their size and resistance to compression in non-anatomical routes, e.g. with external pressure in the subcutaneous tissue and when crossing joints.
- Graft patency tends to be worse than that of the conventional (anatomical) graft because of the required length or external pressures but this may not matter in a patient who is relatively frail and does not have a long life expectancy.
- The number of such grafts is infinite but a few are well recognized and well used and these will be described here.

Axillo-femoral bypass graft[*]

This procedure can be carried out with bilateral axillo-femoral grafts or with a bifurcated graft from one axillary artery supplying both femoral arteries.

Indication for surgery

- Indicated for critical ischaemia secondary to aorto-iliac occlusive disease in patients unfit for aorto-iliac reconstruction.
- Also indicated for revascularization of the lower limbs following removal of an infected aortic graft where the presence of an infected field makes it inappropriate to implant prosthetic material.

Alternatives

- For patients with symptomatic aorto-iliac occlusive disease, the only alternative is aorto-iliac reconstruction after optimization of medical condition.
- For revascularization after removal of an infected aortic prosthesis, the alternative is replacement with another aortic graft with appropriate precautions against further graft infection (see p. 274).

Main risks

- Graft occlusion—early or late.
- Graft infection with risk of pseudoaneurysm formation.
- Compromise of circulation to asymptomatic donor upper limb, including possible steal phenomenon.
- Groin lymph leak.
- Wound infection.

Preoperative work up

- Check the BP in both arms and use the axillary artery on the side of highest pressure. If bilateral axillo-femoral graft is necessary (because the cross-over pathway poses difficulties) and arm pressure is down, duplex the axillary/subclavian artery. If flow is poor here consider angiography with a view to angioplasty to establish good flow before using this as a donor artery.
- FBC.
- Group and save. Cross-match blood if Hb < 10g/dL.
- Clotting screen. Correct if INR > 1.5.
- U & E, creatinine.
- Chest radiograph.
- ECG.

Anaesthesia, preparation, and draping

- GA in most patients.
- Local infiltration of a mixture of quick-acting (e.g. lidocaine) and long-acting local anaesthetic (e.g. bupivicaine or prilocaine) in the very unfit.

---

[*] OPCS codes: L16.1, emergency; L16.2, elective.

- Patient supine on the operating table. Arm on the donor side abducted at 90° on an arm board.
- IV broad-spectrum prophylactic antibiotics.
- Urinary catheter.
- Shave and prepare the skin in both groins and up to the clavicle on the side of the donor artery, extending out to the posterior axillary line and side of the abdomen.
- Drape with both groins and the route from axillary artery to groin exposed, securing drapes with a large transparent adhesive dressing.

Incision and exposure of axillary and femoral arteries
See pp. 212 and 198, respectively.

Procedure

See Fig. 19.1.

1   If the SFA is occluded, the profunda femoris should be dissected to allow clamping distally, facilitating anastomosis on to the proximal profunda artery.

2   The graft (externally supported 8mm PTFE tube graft for axillo-femoral graft and the same material with a side arm of the same size for an axillo-bifemoral graft) is tunnelled subcutaneously between the infraclavicular incision and the two groin incisions using a tunnelling device. The tunnel should lie in the mid-axillary line to reduce the risk of kinking and occlusion of the graft on flexing the trunk. The graft may pass superficial or deep to pectoralis major, depending on how the graft lies best. Tunnelling should be done in a cephalad to caudal direction to minimize the risk of the tunneller traversing the abdominal or thoracic cavities and damaging the organs within. An intermediate incision is made just above the anterior iliac spine to facilitate tunnelling of the limbs of the bifurcated graft to the groin incisions.

3   IV heparin (70u/kg) is administered.

4   After control by application of vascular clamps, longitudinal arteriotomies are made in the axillary artery and both common femoral arteries. If the graft is tunnelled deep to pectoralis major, the arteriotomy in the axillary artery should be on its antero-inferior aspect. If superficial to the muscle, the arteriotomy should be on the antero-superior aspect. When the superficial femoral artery is occluded, the arteriotomy in the common femoral artery can be extended into the origin of the profunda femoris.

5   The graft is anastomosed end-to-side to the axillary artery, using continuous 4/0 or 5/0 Prolene sutures. Clamp the graft close to its origin and restore flow down the axillary artery.

6   The limbs of the graft are anastomosed end-to-side to the common femoral arteries, using 4/0 or 5/0 Prolene sutures. Prior to completion of the anastomoses, the distal vessels are back-bled and the graft unclamped briefly to flush out any clot.

7   The anastomoses are completed and the clamps removed.

9   Both groin wounds are closed in layers, with 2 layer closure of the subcutaneous fascia using 2/0 Vicryl and an absorbable monofilament suture to the skin. Close subclavicular incision with 2/0 Vicryl to subcutaneous tissue and an absorbable subcuticular suture.

Postoperative care

•   Patients are able to mobilize early and are fit for discharge within a few days.

•   There is no evidence supporting graft surveillance in these patients.

Common complications

•   Graft thrombosis is the main complication. Graft thrombectomy is easily carried out with a high success rate for early graft occlusion. It can be performed under local anaesthesia if necessary.

•   Graft infection becomes a problem in those grafts that require repeated thrombectomy.

Morbidity/mortality rates

- Five year primary graft patency is 19–50%.
- Operative mortality is 2–11%.

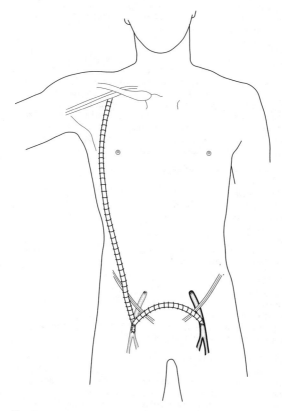

Fig. 19.1 Axillo-bifemoral bypass graft.

Axillo-axillary bypass graft[*]

Indication for surgery Indicated in unilateral proximal subclavian or innominate artery occlusive disease giving rise to arm claudication, digital ischaemia, or posterior cerebral circulation ischaemia. In patients with a subclavian steal syndrome, this procedure may be combined with carotid endarterectomy.

Alternatives

- Short occlusions of the subclavian artery may be amenable to percutaneous transluminal angioplasty.
- In patients fit for thoracotomy with innominate or proximal subclavian occlusion, intrathoracic endarterectomy or reconstruction from the proximal aorta may be performed (usually by cardiac surgeons).
- Reperfusion of the subclavian artery may also be achieved by carotid subclavian bypass or transposition when there is no ipsilateral carotid disease. However, this does carry the risk of neurological events resulting from manipulation of the carotid artery.

Preoperative investigations

- FBC.
- Group and save. Cross-match blood if Hb < 10g/dL.
- Clotting screen. Correct if INR > 1.5.
- U & E, creatinine.
- Chest radiograph.
- ECG.
- Adequate inflow on the donor side may be confirmed by preoperative angiography or duplex ultrasound.

Main risks

- Graft occlusion—early or late.
- Graft infection.
- Wound infection.
- Patients should be warned that the bypass graft may be visible or palpable in a necklace distribution across the neck.

Anaesthesia, preparation, and draping

- GA.
- Local infiltration of long-acting local anaesthetic such as bupivicaine or prilocaine in the very unfit.
- Patient supine with both arms abducted at 90° on arm boards.
- IV broad-spectrum prophylactic antibiotics.
- Shave and prepare the skin from the nipples up to the lower neck and across to the shoulder on both sides.
- Drape to expose the upper chest from clavicles to just above nipples, securing this arrangement with a transparent adhesive drape.

Incision and approach Expose both axillary arteries as on p. 212.

[*] OPCS code L37.1.

Procedure See Fig. 19.2.

1   Tunnel the graft (usually externally supported 8mm PTFE) subcutaneously between the infraclavicular incisions in a shallow U-shape, as a necklace would lie across the neck.

2   Give IV heparin (70u/kg).

3   After control by application of vascular clamps, make longitudinal arteriotomies in both axillary arteries.

4   Anastomose the graft end-to-side to one axillary artery, using continuous 5/0 Prolene sutures. Clamp the graft close to its origin and remove the axillary artery clamps.

5   The anastomosis to the remaining axillary artery is now made, using 5/0 Prolene sutures. Prior to completion of the anastomosis, back-bleed the distal vessel and unclamp the graft briefly to flush out any clot.

6   The anastomosis is completed and the clamps removed.

7   Close both infraclavicular wounds in layers, using 2/0 Vicryl for the subcutaneous fascia and an absorbable monofilament suture for the skin.

Postoperative care
- Patients make a rapid recovery and can normally be discharged from hospital within 24h of surgery.
- There is no evidence to support graft surveillance.

Common complications
- This procedure has a low complication rate.
- Wound infection, graft infection, and graft occlusion are rare.
- Operative mortality is around 2%.

Morbidity/mortality rates Primary and secondary patency rates for axillo-axillary bypass at 10 years are 88% and 91%, respectively. When combined with carotid endarterectomy for steal phenomena, the rates are 86% and 93%.

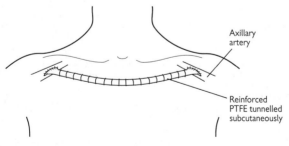

Axillary artery

Reinforced PTFE tunnelled subcutaneously

Fig. 19.2 Axillo-axillary bypass graft.

Femoro-femoral cross-over bypass[*]

Indication for surgery Indicated in critical ischaemia or short distance claudication in the presence of unilateral iliac occlusion. If there is bilateral iliac disease and one side has only a short occlusion or stenosis, that can be dilated before using this artery as the donor vessel.

Alternatives

- Short occlusions of the iliac artery may be amenable to balloon angioplasty ± stent placement.
- In fit patients, aorto-femoral bypass grafting provides higher long-term patency rates.
- Ilio-femoral bypass, either from the contralateral or ipsilateral iliac artery, allows groin dissection to be limited to one side only. Use of the ipsilateral iliac system as donor vessel avoids the risk of compromising the circulation to an asymptomatic limb. Limiting groin dissection to one side reduces the risk of wound infection.

Preoperative investigations

- FBC.
- Group and save. Cross-match blood if Hb < 10g/dL.
- Clotting screen. Correct if INR > 1.5.
- U & E, creatinine.
- CXR.
- ECG.
- ABPIs.

Main risks

- Graft occlusion—early or late.
- Graft infection.
- Compromise of circulation to asymptomatic donor limb, including possible steal phenomenon.
- Groin lymph leak.
- Wound infection.

Anaesthesia, preparation, and draping

- GA ± spinal.
- Spinal anaesthetic.
- Local infiltration of mixture of short-acting (e.g. lidocaine) and long-acting local anaesthetic (e.g. bupivicaine or prilocaine) in the very unfit.
- Patient supine.
- IV broad-spectrum prophylactic antibiotics.
- Urinary catheter.
- Groins shaved and prepared.
- Drapes arranged to expose each groin with a drape to cover the area between them. They are secured with transparent adhesive dressing.

---

[*] OPCS codes: L58.1, emergency; L59.1, elective.

Incision and approach Both femoral arteries are exposed (see p. 198).

Procedure See Fig. 19.3.

1 If either SFA is occluded, the profunda femoris should be dissected to allow clamping distally, facilitating anastomosis on to the proximal profunda vessel.

2 An sc tunnel is formed between the two groin incisions, immediately superficial to the rectus sheath. This is best done with fingers, though a curved aortic clamp may be needed to traverse the fascia in the mid-line. The clamp may then be used to draw a tape through the tunnel to mark it. Care must be taken when forming the tunnel as it is possible to penetrate the bladder with the clamp.

3 IV heparin (70u/kg).

4 Control of the arteries in both groins by applying vascular clamps.

5 Make longitudinal arteriotomies in both CFAs. If the SFA is occluded, the arteriotomy can be extended into the origin of the profunda femoris.

6 A suitable conduit is chosen, depending on the size of the native vessels. In most patients, an 8mm graft is appropriate, although grafts of 6mm or 10mm diameter may be used if the vessels are particularly small or large. Grafts may be of PTFE or Dacron. GSV can be used if there is an infected focus in the leg, if the patient is cachectic and the wounds liable to breakdown or infection, or if previous synthetic cross-over grafts have failed with no obvious problem with inflow or run-off.

7 The graft is introduced into the tunnel, ensuring there is no kinking or twisting. It should lie in a smooth arc within the tunnel and is commonly arranged either as an inverted U-shape, or in sigmoid fashion, depending on how the graft lies in relation to the position of the two arteriotomies.

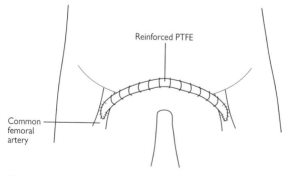

Reinforced PTFE

Common femoral artery

Fig. 19.3 Femoro-femoral cross-over bypass graft.

8   The graft is anastomosed end-to-side to the arteriotomies, using continuous 4/0 or 5/0 Prolene sutures. Prior to completion of the anastomoses, the native vessels are back-bled and the graft flushed to remove any air or clot that has formed.

9   Both groin wounds are closed in layers, with 2 layer closure of the subcutaneous fascia using an absorbable suture.

Postoperative care

There is no evidence that graft surveillance of prosthetic grafts is of any benefit either in terms of maintaining graft patency or preventing limb loss.

Common complications

- Early graft occlusion requires re-exploration of both anastomoses and graft thrombectomy. Technical problems including kinking of the graft must be corrected or re-occlusion is likely.
- Wound infections must be treated aggressively with antibiotics.
- Wound dehiscence that threatens exposure of the prosthetic graft is managed by thorough debridement of all non-viable tissue and wound closure. Where wound closure is not possible, coverage of the graft may be achieved by a sartorius transposition flap.

Morbidity/mortality rates Five-year patency rates of around 70% are expected.

Obturator artery bypass graft[*]

Indication

To revascularize lower limb from aorta or iliac artery to SFA, avoiding the groin because of:

- infection (especially in IV drug abusers and in the femoral end of an aorto-femoral bypass graft). In the case of aorto-femoral graft infection the infected distal limb is removed via the groin after the obturator bypass graft is created, in a separate procedure;
- irradiation damage;
- skin/soft tissue loss due to trauma or tumour resection.

Alternative treatments

- Simple ligation of CFA (± profunda artery and SFA) in patients who present with CFA sepsis (± false aneurysms, ± bleeding). Although the limb is initially fairly ischaemic, in younger patients especially, it rarely reaches a critical level and over the next few days and weeks it improves as collaterals open up. If spontaneous revascularization proves insufficient, then a short synthetic graft can be placed across the groins once sepsis has resolved, although this runs the risk of subsequent graft infection with persistent IV drug abuse in those in whom this is a factor.
- Extra-anatomical bypass graft from contralateral common femoral artery or distal limb of aorto-bifemoral graft to SFA or profunda artery in mid/lower thigh, running sc in the medial thigh to avoid the infected area (usually with synthetic material but vein is also suitable). Infected graft material needs to be removed from the groin, usually prior to creating the new bypass. In the case of an aorto-femoral graft this involves initial division and oversewing of the graft in the uninfected proximal part of the limb via a separate iliac fossa incision and extraperitoneal approach.
- Axillo-SFA bypass graft taking the graft laterally in the groin and then across the mid or lower thigh staying in the subcutaneous plane.
- Where soft tissue cover is lacking, a graft crossing the groin or a repaired native artery can be covered with a sartorius muscle rotation flap (created by dividing sartorius at its proximal attachment to the iliac crest and mobilizing it sufficiently to lay it across the femoral neurovascular bundle without tension). Make sure that all necrotic tissue is debrided from the groin first.

Preoperative work up

- CT scan to assess extent of infection (fluid, oedema, sometimes gas bubbles).
- Arterial imaging (duplex, angiogram, or CTA) to decide on anastomotic sites.
- Cultures of blood and any purulent discharge from the groin or tissue from previous groin debridement to guide prophylactic antibiotic coverage.

[*] OPCS codes: L50.6, emergency; L51.6, elective.

Anaesthesia, preparation, and draping

- GA or epidural.
- IV prophylactic antibiotics based on previous cultures if available; otherwise broad spectrum.
- Urinary catheter.
- Patient supine.
- Shave and prepare ipsilateral lower abdomen and thigh around level of proposed distal anastomosis, leaving the infected groin region covered with a dressing and adhesive dressing.
- Drape to expose separately iliac fossa and thigh, covering the groin with a drape. Secure with a transparent adhesive dressing.

Incision and approach to external iliac artery/proximal limb of aorto-femoral bypass graft

Iliac fossa incision, extraperitoneal approach (see p. 196). For an aorto-femoral graft make your approach to the proximal end of the limb to reduce the likelihood of infection at the anastomosis site.

Incision and approach to distal artery

The site of distal anastomosis is decided on preoperative imaging. For the SFA or profunda artery make a longitudinal incision in medial thigh beyond level of infection. SFA is felt as a relatively superficial firm structure deep to sartorius muscle, which is reflected to allow access. The profunda artery is found at a deeper level through the same incision. If the SFA is occluded and the profunda too small at this level then the graft can be taken down to the popliteal artery (above knee if possible) which is exposed via a more distal medial incision (see p. 200).

Procedure

See Fig. 19.4.

1. Sling the arteries at each anastomosis site. If replacing the distal limb of an aorto-femoral graft check that there is no evidence of infection at this level (poor incorporation of the graft; fluid or pus around the graft). If there is you will need to decide whether to:
   - abandon this approach to bypass grafting and remove the whole of the aorto-femoral graft with extra-anatomic or in line replacement (see p. 272 as for aorto-enteric fistula);
   - abandon bypass grafting altogether and treat with long-term antibiotics; or
   - carry on with an obturator bypass and treat with long-term antibiotics.

   The decision depends on patient fitness and the severity of sepsis.

2. Expose the pelvic aspect of the obturator canal from the upper incision. In IV drug abusers make sure that the external iliac vein and its tributaries are clearly seen as they may be enlarged from arteriovenous fistulae in the groin.

3. Externally rotate the leg. Make a tunnel by passing a tunnelling device from the lower incision, staying deep in the thigh and clear of the infected zone, up through the obturator canal using a finger to enlarge the canal and guide the tunneller. Lay a length of reinforced 6 or 8mm PTFE in the tunnel, removing the tunnelling device.

4. Give IV heparin (70u/kg).

5. If replacing the distal limb of an aorto-femoral graft, divide the graft between clamps and oversew the distal end with 3/0 Prolene.

6. Anastomose the PTFE graft end-to-side to the common or external iliac artery or end-to-end to the proximal limb of the graft with 3/0 Prolene.

7. Anastomose the distal end of the graft end-to-side to the selected distal vessel.

8. Close the wounds with 2/0 Vicryl and 3/0 subcuticular Monocryl.

9. In the case of an infected aorto-femoral graft, once the wounds have been cleaned and dressed, seal them off with transparent adhesive dressing. Remove the drapes and dressings from the groin and reprep and drape this area. Open the groin and remove the graft, closing any arterial defect distally with vein patch or by ligating the common femoral, profunda and SFAs and pulling the divided graft limb down from the pelvis. Wash out with dilute antiseptic solution (e.g. betadine), close deep fascia with 2/0 Vicryl, but leave skin open and pack superficial wound.

Postoperative care

- Continue appropriate antibiotics (based on culture or broad spectrum) for at least 1 week.
- Repack groin wound (after graft removal) at 48h and thereafter every 1–2 days.
- Mobilize on day 1.

Complications
- Bleeding from tunnelling through obturator tunnel. Usually from pelvic surface. Avoid and treat, by getting a clear view of the pelvic surface in this area, enlarging the incision if necessary.
- Early graft obstruction is usually due to poor run-off, kinking of the graft due to excessive length, or compression from an inadequate tunnel.
- Rarely, there is inadvertent routing of the graft into the wall of bladder or vagina. Again avoid by clearly visualizing pelvic route.

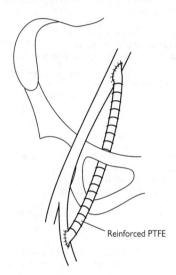

Reinforced PTFE

Fig. 19.4 Obturator bypass graft.

Arteriovenous fistula formation for dialysis*

Indication

Patients who require haemodialysis or are predicted to do so in the near future should be assessed for permanent fistula formation. The alternative is peritoneal dialysis in suitable cases.

Preoperative investigations

Clinical examination alone in the majority of patients is sufficient to determine the choice of access site.

- Arm pulses.
- Visible veins after tourniquet application.
- Scars from previous central cannulation.
- Distended and collateral veins suggesting central obstruction.

If there is suspicion of inadequacy, adjuvant investigations are requested.

- Duplex scanning—arterial and venous.
- Contrast venography (central venous stenosis or occlusion).

There is a hierarchy of preferred sites based on achieving a usable fistula in a convenient location maximizing the length of vein for cannulation. Most surgeons proceed as follows.

- Radiocephalic fistula in non-dominant arm.
- Mid forearm radiocephalic fistula in non-dominant arm.
- Brachiocephalic fistula in non-dominant arm.
- Radiocephalic fistula in dominant arm.
- Mid forearm radiocephalic fistula in dominant arm.
- Brachiocephalic fistula in dominant arm.
- Brachiobasilic fistula in non-dominant arm (with either transposition or tunnelling).
- Brachiobasilic fistula in dominant arm.

When these natural forms of access are exhausted or not suitable then prosthetic grafts are used from the brachial artery either as a loop or straight depending on the outflow vein. The thigh loop based on the femoral vessels is the next option.

Main risks Failure to mature or occlusion is a constant concern. As each site for access is precious and can only be used once it is acceptable to try a more distal fistula even if all the parameters are not optimal. A primary radiocephalic fistula can be expected to be successful in 50–80% of cases.

Procedure

The patient is allowed to increase their dry body weight by 0.5kg for the operation and for 6 weeks after. This helps to prevent dehydration and consequent increase in blood viscosity. If the patient is receiving dialysis the procedure is done on the following day. The veins are marked with application of a tourniquet.

* OPCS code L74.2

Anaesthesia, preparation, and draping
- Local anaesthetic infiltration unless a tunnelling or graft procedure is required in which case GA is required.
- Patient supine with the relevant arm extended on an arm board.
- Arm prepared and draped to expose up to shoulder.

Incision
- Radiocephalic fistula. Longitudinal at the wrist, one-third of the way towards the cephalic vein from the radial artery or oblique. The radial artery is superficial and easily palpated.
- Mid-forearm. Longitudinal, one-third of the way towards the cephalic vein from the radial artery in the forearm. The radial artery lies deeper here between the brachioradialis muscle medially and the flexor carpi radialis muscle laterally; it can often be palpated.
- Brachial fistulas. Transverse in the antecubital skin crease. The brachial artery is deep to the bicipital aponeurosis which is divided. The basilic vein and median nerve are posteriomedial to the artery.
  - For a single-stage brachiobasilic fistula the basilic vein is mobilized along its whole length. It is then disconnected at the cubital fossa end and tunnelled into a subcutaneous position prior to being anastomosed to the brachial artery.

Main steps
1 The artery is exposed over a suitable length, about 2cm. The adjacent vein is exposed and mobilized until it can be offered up to the artery without tension. The vein is disconnected and the distal end tied. A stay suture in the proximal end is useful to prevent orientation errors. A venotomy is made to match the recipient arteriotomy. Some topical papaverine 30mg in 2mL helps to prevent spasm. A soft bulldog clamp may be required to stop troublesome back-bleeding from the vein but, preferably, the weight from an instrument can be used to prevent intimal damage to the vein.
2 Soft bulldog style clamps are applied to the artery. A 1cm arteriotomy is fashioned. The vein is joined to the arteriotomy with 6/0 polypropylene using standard vascular anastomotic technique. Care is taken not to stenose the join and, prior to tying the knot in, inflow may be released to distend the anastomosis. The lie of the vein should be evaluated and further mobilization may be required. A thrill should be palpable in the vein.
3 The wound is closed. The arm is wrapped in gamgee to keep it warm.

Assessment at the end of surgery A bruit should be heard with a stethoscope and a thrill over the anastomosis.

Postoperative instructions The patient may be instructed in the palpation of their fistula to assure themselves it is still running. If concerned they are advised to present to have it checked.

Follow up At 6 weeks the fistula is assessed for maturity, i.e. suitable dilatation of the vein with a good pulsation. The fistula may then be used for dialysis.

Complications
- Wound healing.
- Failure to mature.
  - Inadequate arterial inflow.
  - Competing venous outflow.
- Occlusion.
- Distal arm or hand swelling (arterialization of the veins).
- Distal ischaemia due to arterial steal.
- Aneurysmal dilatation.

Vascular trauma

Limb trauma

Arterial injury in the upper and lower limbs is seen after blunt or penetrating trauma. It is usually associated with other injuries including degloving, soft tissue injury, neurological injury, venous injury, and fractures or dislocations.

Presentation
- External haemorrhage.
- Haematoma.
- Distal ischaemia.
  - Pallor.
  - Reduced temperature.
  - Sensory or motor loss (may be due to nerve injury as well).
  - Absent pulses.
- AV fistula with thrill/bruit.

Initial management
- Resuscitate patient.
- Control external haemorrhage with direct pressure.
- Give analgesia.
- Reduce grossly displaced fractures/dislocations—perfusion may be restored by the reduction.

Investigations
- Blood sampling to determine Hb, baseline renal function, and cross-match blood
- Handheld Doppler or portable duplex can confirm loss of distal flow. Measure ABPI if possible.
- Preoperative angiography may be time-consuming and is rarely necessary to confirm a significant arterial injury. On-table angiography can be performed if required.
- CT angiography may be helpful if CT is required for other injuries but avoid unnecessary delay.

Definitive management
- Consider amputation (usually after discussion with trauma specialists) when limb function cannot be restored because of:
  - non-recoverable neurological injury;
  - extensive bony/ soft tissue injury;
  - loss of viability due to delay in presentation.
- ABPI < 1 is an indication for angiography or exploration (where there is no evidence of chronic ischaemia).
- Single distal vessel injuries without associated ischaemia can be treated with proximal and distal ligation. If both radial and ulnar arteries are transected in the forearm, repair of one vessel is adequate. The dominant artery should be repaired. Dominance can be determined from an Allen's test on the contralateral side.

- The popliteal artery is one of the most commonly injured arteries, usually in association with fracture dislocations around the knee joint (Fig. 20.1).
- A posterior approach using a lazy s incision gives excellent access and facilitates harvesting of the short saphenous vein for bypass. This can be carried out after orthopaedic external fixation.
- Brachial artery injuries are often associated with trauma around the elbow joint and will usually result in ischaemia of the forearm and arm. The injury can generally be bypassed using locally available vein. Forearm fasciotomy including carpal tunnel release should be considered.
- Iatrogenic femoral artery injury resulting from cannulation may result in haematoma or pseudoaneurysm. These can be treated with compression, duplex-guided thrombin injection, coil embolization, or open surgery. Open surgery may involve patch repair or ligation of all vessels as in the case of pseudoaneurysm associated with IV drug abuse.
- Expanding haematoma, or difficult access make open repair challenging. Deployment of a covered stent can deal with many of these injuries. Success has been reported in particular for carotid and axillary artery lesions. Contraindications to stent deployment include:
  - haemodynamic instability;
  - substantial venous injury;
  - insufficient proximal and distal fixation sites;
  - vessel transection.

Where arterial thrombosis has occurred there can be problems with distal embolization or propagation of thrombus and care needs to be taken in these situations.

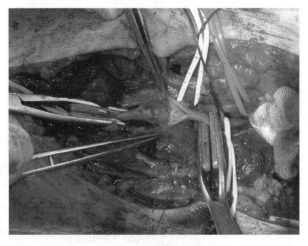

Fig. 20.1 Intimal tear in popliteal artery following trauma.

Anaesthesia and preparation for surgery
- Co-ordinate with orthopaedic/plastic and other specialities.
- GA.
- IV broad-spectrum prophylactic antibiotics.
- Urinary catheter with urimeter bag.
- Use an operating table compatible with on-table angiography.
- Position patient to facilitate exposure of any likely injuries and vein harvest site(s) if required, including contralateral limb. Shave, prepare, and drape accordingly.

Surgery
- Expose the vessel at the site of injury and obtain proximal and distal control.
- Use local heparinization rather than systemic.
- Note associated injuries to veins and nerves.
- Suture repair venous tears in major veins but ligate transections or extensively damaged veins. Vein reconstructions are at high risk of thrombosis because systemic heparinization is usually contraindicated.
- Obtain haemostasis with diathermy/ligation of minor bleeding vessels.
- If major bleeding, uncontrollable locally, consider balloon occlusion or angiographic coiling.
- Wash out wound with warm saline.
- Locate normal artery proximal and distal to the injury.
- Transected arteries may recoil considerable distances and intimal recoil may progress further than the adventitia.
- Assess inflow and run-off by releasing clamps and flushing with heparinized saline.
- Use an arterial shunt if temporizing is required or delay is anticipated, e.g. to stabilize fracture.
- Obtain an on-table angiogram if suspecting further injury or chronic disease.
- If necessary select a more distal site for anastomosis of bypass graft.
- Harvest vein for a conduit. Avoid synthetic material in a potentially contaminated operative field.
- Perform appropriate bypass using inlay, end-to-end, or end-to-side anastamoses.
- Consider fasciotomies.
- Co-ordinate wound closure and dressings with orthopaedic/plastics teams. Ensure at least soft tissue cover of vessels.

Postoperative care
- Standard limb observations with pulse check and Doppler probe insonation if necessary. Record ABPI at least once in postoperative period if possible.
- Check for compartment syndrome, even if fasciotomies were performed (they are sometimes inadequate).
- Monitor urinary output.
- Consider heparin anticoagulation (with great caution) or aspirin.
- Plan wound inspections with delayed closure (3–5 days) of fasciotomies/wounds with or without skin graft.

Management of bleeding

General
- Warm the patient
- Administer clotting factors and platelets
- Consider factor VIIa
- Direct compression
- Duplex-guided thrombin injection

Angiographic
- Balloon occlusion
- Coil insertion
- Covered stent insertion

Surgery
- Pack with large swabs
- Clamp arteries and veins
- Suture/ligate bleeding points
- Balloon occlude artery with Foley catheter

Abdominal vascular trauma

Abdominal vascular injury is found most frequently in association with penetrating trauma but can be associated with blunt trauma such as seat belt injury, significant falls, crush injuries, and pelvic fractures. Major haemorrhage at the time of injury is common but avoid over-recuscitation in an attempt to restore normal BP—it promotes further bleeding and wastes time. Management should be controlled hypotension and rapid transfer to surgery for definitive control of bleeding. Sometimes trauma leads to thrombosis and leg ischaemia at the time of injury. Occasionally vascular damage goes unnoticed at the time and presents later with ischaemia, false aneurysm, or arteriovenous fistula.

Assessment
- Cause of injury.
- Pulse and BP.
- Abdominal distension.
- Femoral pulses.
- Site of penetrating injury.
- External haemorrhage.
- Evidence of pelvic fracture.
- Evidence of spinal injury (especially extension injury).
- Plain abdominal X-ray for gunshot/missile injury to locate site of bullet/metal fragments, etc. is of limited help and should not delay surgery for the unstable patient.
- Angiography is not usually required when there is an obvious vascular injury. It may be useful where an occult injury is suspected in a stable patient, perhaps sometime after the injury.
- CT scan is not indicated primarily for a vascular injury but if undertaken for other reasons may provide some information regarding site of vascular damage.
- Baseline bloods for Hb, U & E, and cross-match blood.

Management
Pelvic fracture with contained retroperitoneal haematoma on CT scan and with good femoral pulses is best managed without vascular exploration. Bleeding is usually tamponaded by the peritoneum and release of tamponade often leads to uncontrollable haemorrhage.

Otherwise, exploratory laparotomy is usually required when there is evidence of a significant intraabdominal bleed. A rapidly deteriorating patient may need an clamp on the lower thoracic aorta via a left thoracotomy in A & E or in theatre to prevent exsanguination. Survival is poor in such cases.

Anaesthesia, preparation, and draping
- GA once patient prepared and draped and surgeons poised to operate; patient can decompensate with GA.
- Keep patient warm and warm all IV fluids.
- Broad-spectrum prophylactic antibiotics IV.

- Large bore IV cannula, central venous and arterial lines (do not use lower limbs for access).
- Cell saver if available.
- Patient supine.
- Shave, prepare, and drape from clavicles to knees in case vein harvest, intrathoracic aortic clamp, or extra-anatomic aortic bypass required.

Surgical principles
- Midline incision from xiphisternum to pubis.
- All haematomas associated with penetrating trauma need exploration except those behind the liver where access is extremely difficult; control here with packing if at all possible.
- If necessary the aorta can be exposed at the diaphragm (see p. 192) and clamped to control bleeding. If this area is surrounded by haematoma, a left thoracotomy and intrathoracic aortic clamp may be required.

In blunt trauma
- Retroperitoneal haematoma in the posterior abdominal wall that is stable, non-pulsatile with an intact peritoneum should not be explored unless it involves the renal hilum (where exploration is debatable—see later) and the duodenum where duodenal perforation needs to be excluded.
- Haematoma in mesentery should not be explored unless the bowel is ischaemic.
- Avoid primary closure of abdominal wall under tension. Increased intraabdominal pressure (which will get worse with bowel oedema and ileus postoperatively) can cause renal failure and respiratory problems. Use mesh closure with moist dressing and take back to theatre for primary closure once abdomen soft and non-distended.

IVC injury
- Commonest intraabdominal vessel to sustain injury.
- When exploration indicated (see above), expose by mobilizing right colon, hepatic flexure, duodenum, and head of pancreas off the posterior abdominal wall.
- Repair with direct closure of tear, PTFE patch, or PTFE interposition graft unless extensive contamination.
- If extensive disruption, can be ligated (especially if patient too unstable to survive major reconstruction).

Aorto-iliac injury
- Intimal tear without evidence of transmural disruption can be managed conservatively.
- In the relatively stable patient aortic dissection or false aneurysm may be treatable by endovascular stenting.
- Surgical exposure of infrarenal aorta and iliacs as on p. 192. Expose suprarenal aorta and its branches by mobilizing left colon, spleen, fundus of stomach, and left kidney over to the right.
- Primary closure is often possible with penetrating trauma.

- If necessary patch or replace disrupted vessel with Dacron or PTFE unless extensive contamination when extra-anatomic bypass may be required.

Mesenteric artery injury

- Primary repair if possible.
- Coeliac axis and its branches can usually be ligated if necessary because of the good collaterals. Liver blood supply can be maintained by the portal vein.
- SMA needs reconstruction rather than ligation.
- Inferior mesenteric artery can usually be ligated.

Renal vascular injury

- Repair of renal artery has relatively poor results with subsequent thrombosis or stenosis leading to hypertension and loss of renal parenchyma. Opinion is divided between advocates of conservative and active management.
- Exploration and reconstruction probably not justified unless it can be performed within 6h of injury. Beyond this kidney is likely to be unsalvageable.
- Expose right kidney by mobilizing right colon, hepatic flexure, duodenum, and head of pancreas off posterior abdominal wall. Expose left kidney by mobilizing left colon, splenic flexure, and spleen over to the right.
- Extensive renal disruption with bleeding warrants nephrectomy.
- Renal artery stenting as delayed treatment is an option in the stable patient.
- Left renal vein can be ligated if repair difficult provided alternative drainage through adrenal, lumbar, and gonadal veins is preserved. If right renal vein needs ligation, nephrectomy is also required because of inadequate alternative drainage.

Postoperative management

- IV fluids and blood as required to maintain renal function and Hb.
- Coagulation may need correction after large blood transfusion.
- Monitor intraabdominal pressure via urinary catheter. An increase above 30cm H_2O is an indication for opening the abdominal wound to release the tension. The wound can be temporarily closed with a synthetic mesh until intraabdominal oedema, haematomas, and ileus resolve.
- Contrast CT where there is strong suspicion of vascular injury that has not been dealt with surgically. In the stable patient, stenosis, flaps, false aneurysms, and arteriovenous fistulae can often be dealt with endovascularly.

Vascular trauma in the neck

The majority of cases involve penetrating trauma in young male adults. Venous injury, especially external jugular, is common. The common carotid artery is the major neck artery most likely to be damaged. Whiplash injury with sudden extension of the cervical spine and with it, stretching of the carotid arteries, is the commonest blunt trauma to cause injury and usually affects the internal carotid artery. Proximal control in common carotid and particularly subclavian trauma may require a thoracotomy.

Assessment
- Cause of injury.
- External haemorrhage.
- BP and pulse.
- Expanding or expansile haematoma.
- Neurological deficit:
  - CNS;
  - cranial nerve;
  - brachial plexus;
  - Horner's syndrome (suggests carotid damage).
- Pain around side of face, ear, or orbit (suggests carotid dissection).
- Difference in arm BPs or other evidence of reduced arm blood flow on affected side (rarely severe even with major subclavian damage because of excellent shoulder collaterals).
- Fracture dislocation of posterior part of 1st rib carries a high probability of subclavian artery disruption.
- Breach in platysma on superficial wound exploration in A & E.

Principles of management
- Immediate surgical exploration is required if patient shows clear evidence of arterial damage:
  - external haemorrhage;
  - haemodynamic compromise not explained by injury elsewhere;
  - expanding or expansile haematoma;
  - arm ischaemia.
- If platysma is intact, surgical exploration in theatre is not required.
- Controversy exists regarding best management of those who fall between these groups. Some advocate exploration of all, others perform angiography or duplex scanning on all to decide on intervention, and a third group advise conservative management with careful monitoring and intervention if relevant signs develop.
- The neck is divided into three zones to guide management (see box).
- Endovascular intervention can be useful in the haemodynamically stable patient to deal with an arterial leak by:
  - proximal balloon occlusion (either as a temporary measure until surgical repair or as a permanent device where surgical access is difficult or impossible, e.g. distal internal carotid artery); or
  - use of a covered stent across the defect.

- Endovascular intervention can be used when complications of unrepaired arterial damage arise later such as dissection, false aneurysm, and arteriovenous fistula.
- Anticoagulation may reduce the thromboembolic complications affecting the brain in carotid and vertebral artery trauma.

Zones of the neck used to guide management of trauma

Zone 1—below a horizontal line 1cm above the clavicle

Zone 2—between zones 1 and 3

Zone 3—between the angle of the mandible and base of skull

Carotid artery

- Penetrating trauma in zone 2 is explored through an incision down the anterior border of sternomastoid (see p. 208).
- Penetrating trauma in zone 1 will probably need proximal control via a median sternotomy.
- Damage from penetrating trauma in zone 3 is difficult to access and may require division of digastric muscle and subluxation or division of the mandibular ramus or balloon occlusion (either a Foley catheter via the surgical wound or as a purely endoluminal approach). Access in zone 3 may be helped by naso- rather than orotracheal intubation by the anaesthetist.
- Repair of penetrating trauma can often be by primary suture. If necessary, synthetic patch, synthetic interposition graft, or transposition of distal ICA to the ECA if there is extensive proximal disruption of the ICA can be performed.
- Damage from blunt trauma (whiplash or crush injury) is often asymptomatic, overlooked at the time, and only diagnosed with onset of CNS signs due to distal embolization from a carotid dissection.
- Blunt trauma may damage both carotid arteries (usually ICAs).
- Unless the artery is bleeding freely after blunt trauma, manage conservatively with anticoagulation for several months. Monitor any progression in this time (duplex or CTA). Endovascular stenting may be helpful for false aneurysms or dissections.

Subclavian artery

- Often associated with brachial plexus and subclavian vein injury.
- Include the anterior chest wall as well as the neck in the sterile operative field to allow for access for proximal control.
- Open the chest and establish proximal control of the subclavian artery before exploring the neck wound. Make a median sternotomy to reach the right subclavian artery and a 'trapdoor' incision (along the 2nd intercostal space, up the sternum, and just above and parallel to the clavicle) to reach the left subclavian artery.
- Alternatively, if the patient is relatively stable, consider temporary balloon occlusion of proximal artery via an endoluminal approach prior to wound exploration to avoid thoracotomy.
- A further alternative is an entirely endoluminal approach with a covered stent placed across the wall defect.

Vertebral artery
- Uncommon injury.
- Can usually be dealt with by occlusion above and below defect through either a surgical or endovascular approach.
- Surgical access is via a supraclavicular approach (p. 210) on to the proximal subclavian artery and the origin of the vertebral artery and via an incision just below the mastoid process to divide sternomastoid and deeper muscles to expose the vertebral artery as it emerges from the transverse process of the 2nd cervical vertebra.
- Anticoagulation may reduce the incidence of neurological sequelae.

Venous injury in the neck If primary repair is not a simple option then ligation is always possible.

Venous surgery

Varicose vein surgery

Venous surgery is rarely life-saving or even limb-saving. Surgery for varicose veins is commonly performed, at least in the UK, but for indications that range from cosmetic concerns in young or middle-aged women to treatment of extensive ulceration in frail elderly patients. Management decisions, as always, need to balance benefit against possible operative morbidity and to consider the full range of non-operative treatments as well (see Chapter 5). Although the surgery is not inherently risky, because the benefits may be less tangible than with arterial surgery, there is more room for patient dissatisfaction. Cosmetic concerns, in particular, are difficult to quantify and only the patient can really say whether the distress caused is worth surgical intervention. It is essential that patients are well informed about possible risks and assured discomfort and restrictions before making their decision. The surgeon must also exercise judgement in this and avoid offering surgery if risk seems out of proportion to any potential benefit.

Indications for surgery

- Varicose veins that are associated with (and likely to be related to) significant symptoms or evidence of complications that cannot be managed satisfactorily by conservative measures (Chapter 5).
  The extent to which this implies 'patient satisfaction' is governed to some extent by the financial restrictions imposed by the prevailing health system.
- Many people have varicose veins that remain entirely asymptomatic throughout their life. The mere presence of varicosities is not an indication for intervention to prevent later problems.
- There is little hard evidence from comparisons of outcomes from surgical versus other treatments for most venous related disease. There is, however, RCT evidence that ulcer healing occurs at a similar rate with surgery and compression bandaging and that the recurrence rate after surgery is lower than that after compression bandaging, provided there is not extensive deep venous reflux.[1]

Alternatives to surgery

- Reassurance.
- Over the counter or prescribed surgical support hose.
- Standard (liquid) sclerotherapy.
- Foam sclerotherapy.
- Ultrasound ablation.
- Laser ablation.

For more discussion see Chapter 5.

Aftercare

- Patients can be discharged later the same day if there are adequate arrangements for transport and home support.
- Simple analgesia, e.g. paracetamol 1g tds plus diclofenac 50mg tds; 3 day supply should suffice.

- Bandages are removed the morning after surgery and replaced with full length compression stockings worn during the day for 2 weeks.
- For 2 weeks after surgery patients are encouraged to walk on a regular basis (for example, at least 5min brisk walking every hour during the day), to raise their feet to at least hip height when seated, and avoid standing still or sitting with the feet down. These restrictions prevent the patient from driving during this time.

Complications

- Haematoma around one of the incisions or along the stripping track. Usually disappears without intervention.
- Wound infection. Usually staphylococcal and settles with a course of oral antibiotics. Very occasionally needs hospital admission for IV antibiotics and perhaps drainage.
- Nerve damage:
  • saphenous nerve injury in GSV surgery, with numbness or tingling on the medial aspect of the calf (approximately 6% incidence);
  • sural nerve damage in LSV surgery, with numbness or tingling in the lateral calf and possibly over the heel (approximately 25% incidence);
  • common peroneal nerve injury in LSV surgery causing foot drop and loss of sensation (uncommon).
  • Most symptoms improve over several months. Numbness (especially if small patch) is no longer noticed even if it persists. Motor injury (common peroneal nerve) requires physiotherapy and ankle support. Nerve conduction studies may be useful in discovering site and extent of injury and documenting any improvement. Specialist referral may be required if more than mild, recovering damage.
- Thread veins. Sometimes appear in the medial thigh; occasionally in the calf following surgery. Cosmetic problem.
- Lymph leakage from the groin. Occasionally after redo groin surgery. Usually settles over a week or so with bed rest (± sc heparin as DVT prophylaxis). Persistent lymph leaks may require re-exploration of the groin wound, ligation of any visible lymphatic vessels, and re-suturing of the wound over a suction drain. The suction drain is left in situ until lymph drainage abates.
- DVT and pulmonary embolus. Known to occur but uncommon (DVT incidence < 5%).

Recurrence of varicose veins after surgery

- Persistence of GSV or LSV after surgery designed to remove them suggests that the main superficial trunk has been wrongly identified. Less likely to happen if stripping.
- There may be a double GSV system. Unless identified before surgery, stripping will remove only one of them and, if the other is incompetent, varicosities will persist.
- True recurrence is often associated with neo-vascularization stemming from the stump of the sapheno-femoral junction. Small, valveless new veins grow down to reconnect with superficial veins in the thigh.

- New varicosities may develop in the other superficial system if only one is treated on the first occasion.
- New varicosities are seen in approximately 30% of patients within 5y and 50% within 25y of GSV stripping and are commoner if only flush ligation of the SFJ is performed.

Greater saphenous ligation and stripping[*]

This operation has become standard surgical practice for the treatment of varicose veins associated with greater saphenous vein (GSV) reflux. It is an extension of the Trendelenburg operation of flush ligation and was initially popularized by Charles Mayo in the early 20th century.

Benefits of stripping
- Reduced need for re-operation.
- Improved venous return through removal of incompetent perforators.

Disadvantages of stripping
In comparison to simple flush ligation of the sapheno-femoral junction, there is:
- increased risk of nerve injury;
- increased complexity of surgery;
- longer operating time;
- increased bleeding.

Preoperative work up
- History and examination; see Chapter 2.
- Diagnosis of sapheno-femoral reflux and incompetence of the GSV can be made on clinical grounds with examination supported by the hand-held Doppler. Ideally all patients should have duplex scanning of the saphenous systems and deep veins to demonstrate areas of reflux, obstruction, and anatomical variants.
- Immediately preoperatively with the patient standing, mark the larger varicosities for avulsion with a skin marker indicating the walls on each side rather than a single line in the middle (which can cause tattooing if the incision is made through it). Mark the GSV at knee level if visible or palpable in case you need to expose it here in order to pass the stripper retrogradely.

Anaesthesia, preparation, and draping
- Usually GA but occasionally patients prefer a spinal.
- Prophylactic broad-spectrum IV antibiotics are advisable if there is significant skin damage or in redo venous surgery.
- Supine with optional head-down tilt.
- Leg board may be used for separation to facilitate access in bilateral cases.
- Shave the medial groin area. Prepare the leg(s) from a few cm above the groin, circumferentially around the limb down to ankle level. Drape to expose the whole limb down to ankle, wrapping a triangulated drape around the foot.

[*] OPCS codes: L87.1; L84.1 (bilateral).

Incision and approach to the sapheno-femoral junction

Make a skin crease incision centred 2.5cm below and lateral to the pubic tubercle. The length of incision depends on the depth of the sapheno-femoral junction (SFJ) but in slim patients 2–3cm is often sufficient. Be prepared to extend the incision if access proves difficult.

Deepen the incision through Scarpa's fascia. There will be a number of veins converging on the GSV before it dives down through a defect in the deep fascia to join the common femoral vein.. Follow these until you find the deep fascial defect and dissect out all the venous tributaries at this point. Treat them with care: in a deep and fatty groin it is possible to mistake the common femoral vein for a superficial tributary. Do not divide any major venous tributaries until you have clearly identified the common femoral vein as a longitudinal structure on the deep aspect of the SFJ, below the deep fascia. Another common mistake when the veins are enlarged is to misidentify the anterior thigh vein or other major tributary as the GSV and its junction with the GSV as the SFJ. Check that what you think is the common femoral vein lies below the deep fascia at the same depth as the common femoral artery.

Procedure

1 Once you have clearly exposed the SFJ, divide all the superficial tributaries, leaving an arterial clip on the peripheral end of the GSV, either absorbable 3/0 ties or Ligaclips on the peripheral ends of the other superficial tributaries, and a single 3/0 tie, suture ligature or clip across the SFJ, being careful not to compromise the lumen of the common femoral vein (Fig. 21.1).

2 Expose the medial and lateral aspects of the common femoral vein and divide (between ties or clips) any tributaries entering at the level of the SFJ (found most commonly on the medial side).

3 Make a short transverse incision in the LSV a centimetre below the clip. Insert the stripper and advance it down the LSV to a few centimetres below the knee joint. Palpate the tip beneath the skin and make a 5mm transverse incision over it in line with the skin crease. Pull the end of the stripper out through this incision, using a medium-sized artery clip if necessary.

4 A sterile inflatable 'roll on' tourniquet, if available, can be rolled up the leg to just below the groin at this point to reduce subsequent blood loss.

5 Pull the stripper down through the vein until the upper end is just above the proximal end of the GSV. If using a Moll stripper, securely tie the proximal end of the LSV to it using one end of a full length 0 Vicryl tie through the hole in the stripper. If using a plastic stripper either tie the vein securely with 0 Vicryl to the stripper just below the slightly expanded end, leaving the full tie length attached, or slip a small stripping head on to the stripper just beyond the vein.

6 The stripper is pulled through to the distal incision with the vein attached. If the GSV tears so that only part is retrieved, use the length of attached Vicryl lying within the stripping pathway to pull the Moll 'retriever' (or the plastic stripper with a head attached to its upper end this time) down the same pathway to remove the remnant. In case this fails, attach a further full length tie to the upper end of the retriever or stripper so that this then marks the pathway. If necessary this can be tied to the reversed retriever or plastic stripper + head at the distal end, after dividing the GSV at this point and the vein stripped upwards. See Fig. 21.2. If a significant length of GSV still remains in the thigh despite these attempts to remove it, it can be avulsed through a series of small skin crease incisions over it.

7 The remaining LSV distal to the stripper may be avulsed or tied.

8 Avulsions of prominent varicosities (see p. 458) is often performed in conjunction with GSV stripping.

9 Manual compression is applied to the mid-thigh and distal wounds to achieve haemostasis.

10 Close the groin with 2/0 Vicryl to Scarpa's fascia and a 3/0 absorbable subcuticular suture.

11 Infiltrate the groin wound with bupivicaine or other long-acting LA.

12 Close the distal skin incision with a single subcuticular suture.

13 Clean the limb. Apply a pad over the distal incision and a crepe bandage from toes to upper thigh. Remove the tourniquet at this stage, rolling it over the bandage.

Tips for passing the stripper

- Check duplex for LSV course if available.
- Use a Roberts clamp attached to the proximal end to rotate the tip.
- Guide passage of stripper with manual compression on thigh.
- Substitute plastic for metal stripper and vice versa.
- Locate vein distally through small incision and pass stripper upwards.

Management of substantial bleeding from the femoral vein
See p. 226.

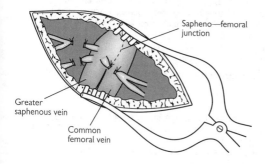

Fig. 21.1 Sapheno-femoral ligation.

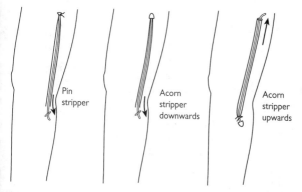

Fig. 21.2 Manoeuvres to strip the GSV.

Flush ligation of sapheno-femoral junction[*]

This can be done under local anaesthetic infiltration of the groin and so is useful in frail patients with significant problems related to venous disease that cannot be treated by other means. Such patients may have a relatively short life expectancy so that durability of the procedure (in comparison to high saphenous ligation with stripping) is not a major issue.

Anaesthesia, preparation, and draping

- Local infiltration (mark a line in the skin crease centred over a point 2.5cm below and lateral to the pubic tubercle, 3–4cm long and infiltrate along it with a mixture of short- and long-acting anaesthetics), spinal or GA.
- Shave and prepare the groin.
- Place drapes around the groin area.

Incision and approach
As for 'High saphenous ligation and stripping' (p. 449).

Procedure

1. As for 'High saphenous ligation and stripping', step 1, but ligate or Ligaclip the GSV as well, if possible removing 2–3cm of it to separate the stump from the SFJ.
2. Close the groin with 2/0 absorbable suture to Scarpa's fascia and subcuticular 3/0 absorbable suture.
3. Apply a full length support stocking unless the lower leg has a bulky compression bandage in place in which case no further compression is required.

[*] OPCS codes: L85.1; L84.1 (bilateral).

Lesser saphenous vein ligation and stripping*

Lesser saphenous incompetence is found in about 15% of patients with varicose veins. The LSV lies deep to the deep fascia for most of its course and is therefore less visible than the GSV. Incompetence is easily missed on clinical examination unless you palpate specifically over the course of the vein in the posterior calf. LSV incompetence is associated with lateral gaiter area ulcers.

Preoperative work up
- Clinical assessment (Chapter 2).
- Duplex marking of sapheno-popliteal junction (SPJ).
- Consent. Make sure that the patient is aware of the possibility of nerve damage (as well as other risks). See p. 445.

Anaesthesia, preparation, and draping
- GA (or spinal or local infiltration if necessary).
- Patient prone.
- Posterior calf shaved.
- Skin prepped from 3–4cm above duplex-marked SPJ down to ankle on posterior, medial, and lateral aspects (or circumferentially if anterior varicosities or perforators to be dealt with and no plans to turn the patient for GSV surgery).
- Drape to expose back and sides of calf.

Incision and approach to sapheno-popliteal junction
- Transverse incision at level of duplex marked SPJ.
- Deepen incision through deep fascia and place a self-retaining retractor on the edges of the fascia.
- Look for the LSV running longitudinally and trace it upwards until it dips down towards the popliteal vein. Follow it down, taking care not to damage the sural or common peroneal nerves, until you reach the SPJ. You may find the superficial continuation of the LSV (the Giacomini vein) joining it before it dips down. A tributary from the soleal sinuses often joins the LSV just distal to the SPJ but is much smaller than the SPJ and unlikely to be confused with it (Fig. 21.3).
- If the LSV is not obvious in the fat of the popliteal fossa despite extensive superficial dissection you have two options. Either:
  - make a small transverse incision in the midline below your current incision and find the LSV deep to the deep fascia at this level. Open the vein and pass a stripper up so that it can be palpated in the original incision to locate the LSV; or
  - feel for the popliteal pulse and dissect down on to the artery. Find the popliteal vein adjacent to the artery and locate the SPJ from the level of the duplex marking.

---

* OPCS codes: L87.2, ligation + stripping; L85.2, ligation only; L84.2, bilateral ligation ± stripping.

Procedure

1 Dissect out the SPJ (watching out for the sural nerve) and divide it between a tie of 2/0 absorbable braided suture on the popliteal vein side, taking care not to narrow the deep vein, and a clip on the LSV end.

2 Mobilize the LSV to the lower wound margin. Make a transverse venotomy and pass down a short Moll stripper or a plastic stripper. The end of the stripper will be palpable in the mid to lower calf, passing laterally as it descends. Make a short vertical incision over the tip and pull it out until the top end of the stripper lies just above the proximal end of the vein.

3 Tie the end of the stripper firmly to the proximal end of the vein with a 0 braided tie.

4 Pull the stripper out from the distal wound.

5 The LSV can be fragile and fail to strip out. Rather than risk the sural nerve with repeated attempts to remove the residue, remove any remnant of vein accessible under direct vision from your proximal incision. This will at least reduce the risk of recurrence.

6 Close the popliteal fossa with 2/0 absorbable braided suture to the deep fascia and a subcuticular absorbable 3/0 monofilament suture.

7 Infiltrate the wound with long-acting LA.

8 Apply pads to the wounds and a crepe bandage from toes to upper calf.

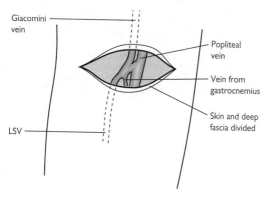

Fig. 21.3 Exposure of the sapheno-popliteal junction.

Ligation of incompetent perforator veins[*]

There is some debate as to whether this is necessary routinely. Duplex scanning often reveals incompetent perforators that are not evident clinically and would otherwise be left untouched with no obvious detriment to outcome. Stripping of the main superficial trunk alone has been shown to restore competence to perforators in some cases. Where an incompetent perforator appears to be feeding a major group of varicosities in isolation from the main trunk, division of the perforator can certainly be justified. Perforator ligation is often combined with truncal surgery, however, on the basis that everything possible should be done on the first operation to prevent recurrence and the need for reintervention.

Preoperative work up Mark site of incompetent perforator using duplex immediately prior to surgery.

Anaesthesia, preparation, and draping As for truncal surgery (see p. 448) with the patient either prone or supine depending on site of perforator.

Procedure

1   Make a skin crease incision about 1cm long, centred on the duplex-guided mark.
2   Deepen the incision to search for a superficial vein that will lead to the perforator. Dissect out the vein until a deep tributary is found that penetrates the deep fascia.
3   Divide the perforator vein between 2/0 absorbable braided ties or Ligaclips.
4   If the perforator vein cannot be found, sweep the deep fascia with you finger to seek the perforator vein crossing it. You may disrupt it with your finger if it is small but otherwise ligate and divide it.
5   Close the wound with subcuticular 3/0 monofilament absorbable suture.

[*] OPCS code L85.8.

Avulsion of varicose veins[*]

This is a cosmetic procedure, often combined with truncal surgery.

Preoperative work up On the day of surgery, mark the most obvious varicosities with the patient standing. Use a water resistant skin marker to indicate both edges of the vein: a central mark may lead to tattooing.

Anaesthesia, preparation, and draping As for truncal surgery (see p. 448) with the patient either prone or supine depending on site of perforator.

Procedure

1. Use a no. 11 blade to make a short stabbing incision in the direction of the skin crease over the varicosity as marked.
2. Use a vein hook or a pair of fine Mosquito clips to pick up the edge of the vein and ease it out of the wound. Gently tease off any adherent connective tissue and cutaneous nerves until the full width of the vein is visible. Divide it between clips.
3. Using the attached clip pull the vein out of the wound for 2–3cm if possible. Place another clip across the vein as it disappears under the skin edge and pull again, reapplying a clip further along if necessary. The vein will break at some point. You may be able to retrieve the distal end from under the skin edge and pull out some more. It is not necessary to remove the entire length of a varicosity. Interrupting it at several points works just as well in the long run.
4. Close the wound with a Steristrip.

Surgery for recurrent varicose veins[*]

Indication for surgery Clinically significant recurrence of varicose veins is common. Long-term follow-up studies have demonstrated recurrence in 30% of patients by 5y. Though the indications for surgery are similar to those for primary varicose veins, there should be a higher threshold for offering surgery, as the risks of complications are greater. Many of the recurrences are due to neovascularization originating from the stump of the SFJ, which connects to thigh veins and leads to reflux down the limb.

Preoperative investigations

- All patients should be assessed preoperatively with duplex ultrasonography, as the pattern of recurrence cannot be accurately assessed by clinical examination. Coexistent deep venous incompetence or occlusion can also be excluded.
- It is imperative that patients undergoing re-do surgery on the lesser saphenous system have the sapheno-popliteal junction and LSV marked using duplex ultrasound preoperatively.
- In patients undergoing surgery for recurrent GSV incompetence, it may be useful to have the GSV in the thigh marked preoperatively, particularly if the recurrence does not extend up to the groin.

Alternatives

- Recurrent superficial varicosities in the absence of any truncal reflux demonstrated on duplex ultrasonography may be treated with liquid sclerotherapy alone.
- Where recurrent truncal reflux has been demonstrated, this may be suitable for treatment with one of the newer non-surgical interventions (see Chapter 5).

Anaesthesia, preparation, and draping

- As for primary surgery.
- Broad-spectrum prophylactic antibiotics are probably indicated given the higher risk of wound infection, especially with groin re-exploration.

Procedure

Recurrence in greater saphenous system

In patients in whom a recurrent SFJ has been demonstrated on duplex ultrasound, the SFJ should not be approached through scar tissue from the previous operation.

[*] OPCS codes: L85.3, ligation; L84.4, bilateral recurrent GSV; L84.5, bilateral recurrent LSV; L84.6, recurrent GSV and LSV.

1   Make an incision about 1cm above the previous groin incision,
    curving down medially. Deepen the incision until the inguinal liga-
    ment is exposed and find the common femoral vein as it passes
    underneath it. If there is any difficulty in finding it, feel for the femo-
    ral pulse and expose the anterior surface of the CFA at the inguinal
    ligament. Find the common femoral vein on its medial side.
2   Continue dissection caudally along the front of the common femoral
    vein until the stump of the SFJ, with its leash of new veins, is encoun-
    tered. The junction is carefully dissected out until freed on all sides.
    It can then be divided between artery forceps and transfixed.
3   Where duplex has demonstrated the presence of a residual GSV
    extending from the groin this can now be stripped to just below the
    knee as in primary varicose veins.
4   The cribriform and subcutaneous fascia are closed with a braided
    absorbable suture. The skin is closed with an absorbable
    monofilament suture.
5   In patients in whom there has been found to be a residual GSV in
    the lower thigh giving rise to varicosities in the absence reflux from
    the SFJ, the GSV can be ligated at its proximal end and then stripped
    down to knee level. It is useful in this situation if the vein has been
    marked using duplex ultrasound preoperatively.

Recurrence in lesser saphenous system

Recurrent reflux in the LSV is sometimes due to failure to reach the SPJ
in the first operation. The LSV is tied off, and perhaps stripped, some
distance below the junction and the reflux in the proximal system
extends back down into the lower leg as new tributaries develop. Duplex
reveals an SPJ some distance above the scar. In this case surgery is relatively straightforward and proceeds as for primary ligation and stripping,
although it is unlikely that much can be stripped and it may be better just
to remove as much LSV from under the wound edge as you can reach.

Where recurrent reflux in the lesser saphenous system has been
shown on preoperative duplex assessment, with neovascularization from
a ligated junction, the potential benefits of attempted flush ligation of a
recurrent SPJ are probably out-weighed by the risks of damage to
neurovascular structures inherent in re-exploration of a scarred popliteal
fossa.

1   A small transverse incision is made over the marked LSV as
    proximally as possible whilst avoiding the previously operated field.
    The deep fascia is exposed and incised along the line of its fibres.
2   The LSV is exposed and carefully dissected free of adjacent
    structures. Special attention is given to identifying the sural nerve,
    which may be adherent to the vein and dissecting it off the vein
    atraumatically.
3   The vein is divided between artery forceps. The proximal end is
    ligated or transfixed as high as possible and the distal end is stripped
    to the lower calf if possible. If it will not strip, remove as long a
    length as possible from under the wound edge.
4   The deep fascia is reconstituted with a braided absorbable suture
    and the skin closed with a 3/0 absorbable monofilament suture.

5 Recurrent superficial varicosities may be removed by multiple avulsions in the usual way.
6 Crepe bandages are firmly applied over gauze pads placed along the line of the GSV and over the sites of avulsions.

Surgery for deep venous disease

Extensive reflux in the deep veins may be postthrombotic or develop in much the same way (although much less commonly) as superficial venous incompetence with no previous thrombosis. In either case it is associated with significant morbidity in terms of leg swelling and skin damage, including ulceration. Reflux at popliteal level appears to cause most damage and there have been extensive attempts to replace or repair the valves at this point in order to restore competence. In the postthrombotic limb this is usually unsuccessful. In the non-thrombotic limb there has been limited success in specialist centres but such surgery is beyond the scope of this handbook. Most patients with extensive deep venous reflux are treated with compression hose successfully.

Most DVTs recanalize and largely disappear but some persist. If there is significant outflow obstruction to the leg the patient will experience leg swelling, discomfort, and skin breakdown. This is usually managed with class 3 full length compression hose but sometimes this fails to halt significant discomfort and skin damage. In such circumstances it may be worth investigating with a view to improving venous drainage. Venous duplex combined with MR venography (or conventional venography if MRV not available) will show the extent of occlusion and development of collaterals. Most of these patients have iliac vein thrombosis. You need to know the following.

- Is the common femoral vein occluded?
- Does the IVC or other iliac vein also contain thrombus?
- Is there thrombus or reflux in the contralateral deep veins or GSV?
- Is there good collateralization around the occlusion?

Drainage that has to go through poor collaterals can probably be improved by intervention. If the collaterals are good, the risk is that they will occlude when drainage via an alternative route is established but, if that alternative then fails, the leg may be worse than it was initially.

The surgical option is a Palma operation. The radiological alternative is stenting of the occluded iliac vein.

- Both require an ipsilateral patent common femoral vein.
- Both require an open IVC.
- Surgery also needs a patent and competent contralateral GSV that is superfluous to requirements. If there has been thrombotic deep vein occlusion in the contralateral leg, the GSV may be an important means of venous drainage and should not be removed.
- Surgery also needs a patent contralateral iliac vein.

Neither procedure is guaranteed to last. Surgery has a longer track record and is probably more successful but there have been no trials directly comparing the two procedures. The patient will still have to wear compression on the affected leg.

Palma operation*

This operation involves mobilization of the contralateral GSV for use as a subcutaneous cross-over graft to divert venous drainage to the contra-lateral iliac system (Fig. 21.4). The competent valves in the GSV are important in preventing reflux into the affected leg.

Preoperative work up
- Venous investigations (see p. 464).
- Duplex marking of contralateral GSV is useful.

Anaesthesia, preparation, and draping
- These patients are at high risk for DVT and pulmonary embolus. Give prophylactic sc heparin injection prior to surgery (they will probably be fully anticoagulated postoperatively).
- GA or spinal (you do not want to interrupt anticoagulation postoperatively to remove an epidural catheter).
- Prophylactic broad spectrum antibiotics.
- Shave and prep both groins, the suprapubic region, and the contralateral leg circumferentially down to knee level.
- Drape to expose these areas.
- Dissect out the contralateral GSV down to knee level without dividing the SFJ or distally. Divide and ligate or clip tributaries.
- Dissect out the ipsilateral common femoral vein and gently sling it at the inguinal ligament.
- Make a subcutaneous tunnel with a curved aortic clamp between the two groin wounds. Measure the length of graft required using a thick tie between clips.
- Divide the contralateral GSV to give the required length from the SFJ. Ligate the distal end.
- Tunnel the graft across. Anastomose it end-to-side to the common femoral vein using 5/0 or 6/0 Prolene suture.
- Flow through the graft can be improved by creating a temporary arteriovenous fistula in the ipsilateral groin. Find one of the minor arterial branches of the ipsilateral common femoral artery, divide it about a cm from the femoral artery, spatulate the end, and anastomose it end-to-side to the hood of the graft. Lay a silk tie loosely around this fistula and knot the ends together several cm from the fistula. Bury the ends of this tie within the subcutaneous tissues of the wound.
- Close the wounds with 2/0 braided absorbable suture to Scarpa's fascia and 3/0 subcuticular absorbable monofilament suture.

Postoperative care
- Full anticoagulation with heparin iv/sc (iv may be easier to control if re-operating to close temporary fistula) for 2 weeks unless converting back to long-term warfarin (after closure of temporary fistula).
- Full length class 3 compression hose on affected leg.
- Mobilize the following day.
- Duplex scan of graft to check flow within 48h.

* OPCS code L83.1.

Closure of temporary fistula

This can be performed about a week after the initial surgery provided flow across the graft is good. If it is not good (or has occluded) then you may decide not to ligate the fistula.

Under GA (or LA infiltration if necessary) the ipsilateral groin is prepared and draped. The skin suture is removed and the silk tie located in the subcutaneous tissues. The ends are drawn tight and followed down, opening up Scarpa's fascia to expose the region of the fistula. Tie the ligature firmly around the fistula; it does not need to be dissected out cleanly but ensure that no other important structures lie within the tie. Close the wound as before. Check flow in the graft with duplex postoperatively.

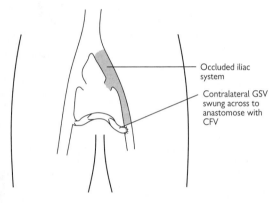

Occluded iliac system

Contralateral GSV swung across to anastomose with CFV

Fig. 21.4 Palma operation to provide alternative venous drainage when iliac vein is occluded.

Reference

1 Barwell JR, Davies CE, Deacon J, *et al.* (2004). Comparison of surgery and compression with compression alone in chronic venous ulceration (ESCHAR study); randomized controlled trial. *Lancet* **363**, 1854–9.

The future of vascular surgery

Effects of an ageing population on future health care

We face an era of ageing population, but a population that has increasing expectations of medicine, society, and their own activity. At the same time the relative reduction in the younger age group will diminish the social resources available to look after the elderly, either as family or paid employees.

The cost of hospital care increases with its complexity and the only way in which we will be able to afford care of the elderly, be it for vascular disease or other problems, is, firstly, to promote lifestyle modifications that reduce the risk of vascular disease more effectively and, secondly, to promote non-surgical management strategies in the community. A major reduction in the percentage of the population who smoke has enormous potential to reduce the burden of vascular disease. Expertise in vascular disease management needs to be developed within the community in GPs, nurses, physiotherapists, and other community carers within a network that includes secondary care primarily as an advisory and only occasionally as a direct patient resource. Patients themselves need to take a lead in recognizing health risk and the onset of health problems and taking responsibility for their own well-being.

Secondary and tertiary care need to concentrate at the sophisticated end of health-care delivery, which demands expensive radiological, surgical and intensive care support for the select group of patients who require it. This highly specialized care should not be diluted by demands for other care that could be provided equally well (and perhaps more efficiently) in the community. This is not to diminish secondary care's role but rather to enhance it by making it part of a wider network with the community in providing health care. The fact that much of its role in the community may be largely advisory does not diminish its importance.

Increasing age inevitably invites atherosclerotic disease as part of the degenerative process. Staving off that disease depends on modifications to diet, physical activity, and smoking habits and, in some individuals, the addition of medication to lower BP, glucose, and cholesterol. Advances in drug therapy will no doubt result in powerful drugs that can dissolve atheroma. This may abolish much of vascular surgery and radiology but, on the other hand, may lead to more aneurysmal and embolic disease.

Vascular investigations

Smaller, more portable, and cheaper duplex equipment is becoming available. The quality of image production and analysis is improving all the time and it seems likely that the vascular surgeon of the future will carry this equipment in their pocket and use it routinely as an adjunct to the clinical examination. It also opens up the possibility that some of this technology will transfer to the community, perhaps in a simpler form, for initial investigation of vascular patients and for population screening. Early detection of atherosclerotic disease (even as early as increased intima-medial thickness) could be used to target interventions more effectively and feed into the reduction of vascular disease burden.

Treatment of vascular disease

Radiological techniques will no doubt play an increasing part in the treatment of vascular disease. Endovascular aortic stenting will become the mainstay of aneurysm repair and technology will overcome problems with access and endoleaks. Medication is likely to reduce the volume of atherosclerotic disease and the generation of thrombus within the circulation. When patients do present with occlusive disease, no doubt better stents will be developed that resist thrombosis and intimal hyperplasia and remain patent even in low flow situations down the leg. Adding to this the possibility that growth factors will be used to develop and repair the microcirculation, it is difficult to see a major role for open vascular arterial surgery in the longer term apart, perhaps, from its use in trauma. Venous disease is also likely to disappear from operating lists as minimally invasive techniques such as foam sclerotherapy take over. In the future one might envisage endovascular placement of venous stents with good long-term patency and, perhaps, synthetic deep venous valves.

The vascular surgeon

The surgeon of the future, whatever their speciality, needs to be a physician who can operate. The vascular surgeon, in particular, also needs to be capable of manipulating an endovascular catheter in the X-ray suite. The rapidly changing face of vascular surgery means that surgeons cannot afford to be 'merely' highly specialized technicians. They need to maintain a broader view of patient care and take a lead in developing new aproaches to improve on outcome for their patients rather than concentrating on preserving their own surgical practice.

Index